GET WELL WITH
THE HAY DIET

Food Combining and Good Health
with more help for
medically unrecognised illness

JACKIE HABGOOD

SOUVENIR PRESS

First published 1999 by Souvenir Press Ltd,
43 Great Russell Street, London WC1B 3PA

Reprinted 1999
Reprinted with updating 2003

ISBN 0 285 63535 2

Typeset by Rowland Phototypesetting Ltd,
Bury St Edmunds, Suffolk
Printed in Great Britain by
Creative Print and Design Group (Wales), Ebbw Vale

To those whose many genuine complaints are
being dismissed as 'all in the mind', but who may well be
suffering needlessly from the current epidemic of medically
unrecognised illness, unaware that simple and
effective treatment exists

To those who do not think of themselves as ill, but would
like to feel better

To slimmers who cannot lose weight however little they eat

To the many people who feel unaccountably tired and stressed

To those whose health is poor despite a healthy diet

To anyone who feels constantly ill and cannot find out why

To anyone with unexplained mental and nervous problems
which do not respond to conventional medicine

To anyone wishing to reduce their dependence on
prescription drugs

To those with any problem at all which conventional
medicine believes you have to live with

And to those who have tried both conventional
and complementary medicine but whose
problems stubbornly persist

I dedicate this book

ABOUT THE AUTHOR

Jackie has been a 'medical mystery' for most of her life. Conventional medicine provided few answers and little help, hence this book. Now largely recovered, she shares what she has learnt along the way. Jackie trained as a nurse, midwife and health visitor. She works as a counsellor in health awareness and lectures widely. This is her second book. Her first, *The Hay Diet Made Easy*, introduces the diet. This book is a follow-up for those who need more help.

Acknowledgements

My love and thanks go to Ken, Chloe and Alexandra who helped to make this book possible. My thanks again to the growing number of doctors and dietitians who are opening their minds to the approach I describe in these pages. And many thanks to those who have so generously shared their experiences.

J.H.

Contents

Note to Readers

Every care has been taken to ensure that the instructions and advice given in this book are accurate and practical. However, where health is concerned—and in particular a serious problem of any kind—I must stress that there is no substitute for seeking advice at the earliest available opportunity from a qualified medical practitioner. All persistent symptoms, of whatever nature, may have underlying causes that need, and should not be treated without, professional elucidation and evaluation. It is therefore very important, if you intend to use this book for self-help, only to do so in conjunction with duly prescribed conventional or other therapy. In any event, read the advice carefully, and pay particular attention to the precautions and warnings both general and specific.

The Publisher makes no representation, express or implied, with regard to the accuracy of the information and/or advice contained in this book, and legal responsibility or liability cannot be accepted by the Author or the Publisher for any errors or omissions that may be made or for any loss, damage, injury or problems suffered or in any way arising from following the advice offered in these pages.

Jackie Habgood
June 1999

Preface

A sick person is seldom asked exactly what he is eating or drinking. Anyone who does ask, as I do, receives some surprising replies and it becomes immediately obvious why that person is ill. So here is a simple introduction to what you can achieve by changing your diet. It is based on an understanding of how the body works and how we can work with it to assist our own recovery. There is so much more you can do for yourself if you are willing to work hard on your diet.

It was my own battle with chronic illness that led me to investigate my diet. For thirteen years I felt so exhausted and ill I hardly knew how to get through the day. I was hooked on antidepressants, and doctors could not help. Had I been more aware of the effects of food, and the potential danger from mercury amalgam dental fillings, I could never have let myself deteriorate for so long. I would have come to the aid of my exhausted body right from the start; I would have given it my full support if only I had known exactly how to do it.

This book will help those who are constantly under par or who are deteriorating mentally and physically and do not understand why. Most people in this situation are suffering from common complaints which all respond to a few simple changes in diet, and the results can sometimes be spectacular. This book will help you identify your condition, show you how you can help yourself and tell you where to get further help if you need it. If you are a problem slimmer, you will find that the Hay diet and blood sugar control can often work where all else has failed.

During the years I was ill I thought that if the doctor could not help, then nobody could. I believed that if there had been any other way to recover, he and I would have known about it.

11

Neither of us suspected for a moment that so many powerful alternatives existed. I have found so many things I could do to help myself that I have never run out of ideas. Today I wake before six, I am busy all day and I feel well. Information like this is hard to come by, and I have pieced it together gradually over several years. Naturally I could have recovered faster if someone had presented me with it all in one book like this. I hope you will find it all as helpful and exciting as I have, and that it will change your life as it has changed mine.

Lastly, if you have a Hay diet success story to tell I would be delighted to hear it. Contact me on email: jackiehabgood@ zetnet.co.uk

Or visit my Website: http://www.users.zetnet.co.uk/ habgood

J.H.

Introduction

Tired of being tired? So many of us are mysteriously tired and stressed these days that we hardly consider it unusual any more and struggle on in the mistaken belief that nothing can be done about it. Yet everyday tiredness is easy to relieve—anyone can do it. You can recover much of your strength and stamina, often in quite a short space of time.

Do you suffer from chronic fatigue?
Some people have become so exhausted that life is all work and no play. Others are ill in bed for long periods and are desperate for an explanation of their many symptoms. They have had every conceivable test and examination, but most prove negative. They have been to specialists, they have taken prescribed drugs, had operations, but nothing helps very much. Many have tried complementary medicine, too, and got nowhere. People who just want to get on with their lives are having to put their plans on hold while they struggle through the day. Yet even they can often find considerable relief, sometimes in a matter of weeks.

M.E. (Myalgic Encephalomyelitis)
This devastating neurological illness is often associated with a virus infection, and characterised by exercise-induced fatigue. There is extreme mental and physical exhaustion, undue muscle fatigue and pain, and many other symptoms which fluctuate unpredictably. It is a complex condition and there are no simple answers, but the information in this book will be of tremendous help.

Not all in the mind

A long list of mental and physical symptoms is often put down to stress and doctors can do little to help, being unaware of the swift and powerful effects of changes in diet. Yet in recent years there has been a revolution in the treatment of nervous problems in particular. Even mental illness can now be speedily improved by using simple but powerful nutritional methods, and also by freeing the body of its burden of mercury. Body and mind recover together, automatically.

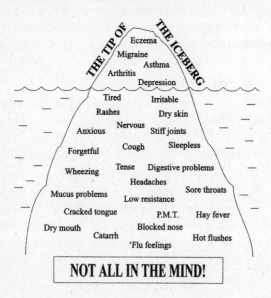

THE TIP OF THE ICEBERG

Eczema
Migraine
Asthma
Arthritis
Depression

Tired — Irritable
Rashes — Dry skin
Anxious — Nervous — Stiff joints
Forgetful — Cough — Sleepless
Wheezing — Tense — Digestive problems
Headaches
Mucus problems — Low resistance — Sore throats
Cracked tongue — P.M.T. — Hay fever
Dry mouth — Blocked nose
Catarrh — Hot flushes
'Flu feelings

NOT ALL IN THE MIND!

MEDICALLY UNRECOGNISED ILLNESS

Low blood sugar, candida and food intolerance are very common conditions which are at present medically unrecognised, but fortunately they, too, rapidly respond to changes in diet, so there is much you can do to help yourself.

LOW BLOOD SUGAR

This is by far the most common cause of everyday tiredness, and the most easily relieved. It is our greatest health problem, and a major cause of nervous and emotional disorders, too. Few of us realise what low blood sugar can lead to when it is neglected. It plays an important part in chronic illness of many kinds.

CANDIDA

This debilitating yeast or thrush infection is extremely common and becoming more widespread. Usually it begins in the bowel or the vagina, and unless it is treated systemically in the early stages it can spread throughout the body, producing an ever-growing list of mysterious mental and physical symptoms. There is a diet designed to starve the yeast and there are many ways of strengthening your natural resistance to it. Powerful antifungal drugs and natural fungicides are also widely available. It can usually be vastly relieved in a matter of weeks.

FOOD INTOLERANCE

Many people cannot understand why they are constantly run down and unaccountably stressed, despite a healthy diet. Intolerance to natural foods is extremely common but seldom recognised. Removing troublesome foods from the diet can bring fast and powerful relief from a great variety of problems, and again the results can sometimes be spectacular.

MERCURY POISONING (FROM SILVER, GREY OR BLACK METAL FILLINGS)

Mercury leakage from amalgam dental fillings is seriously affecting many people, and concern is growing worldwide. Amalgam fillings are 50 per cent mercury, which has long been known to be highly poisonous, and very many people are also hypersensitive to it. It is frequently involved in mental and neurological disorders and can cause a multitude of other medical problems. Replacing mercury with white fillings can bring huge and speedy relief, sometimes with dramatic results. The Hay diet is a cleansing diet which further assists the body to dispose of its burden of mercury. There is more information in chapter 16.

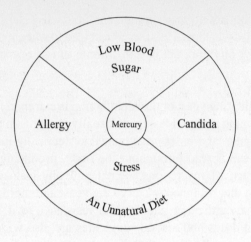

THE ROOTS OF ILLNESS

MYSTERY ILLNESSES
Mystery illnesses of all kinds respond readily to the Hay diet and the other natural healing methods described in this book, even where no diagnosis can be made, because they put the body in a position to right itself. Problems which baffle medical minds do not so easily defeat the wisdom of the body.

WHAT IS THE HAY DIET?
It is supernutrition, a nature cure, and you are on the mend from the moment you begin it. It can work for so many problems because it triggers and supports a continuous process of natural healing, gradually restoring normal function to every organ in the body as far as is possible. Given the right food the body soon gets to work repairing everything that needs mending. It works on your general health, on every part of you, and whole catalogues of symptoms frequently disappear together. Much more can be done for most illnesses than many of us realise.

Dr William Hay (1866–1940)

Dr Hay was an American, and during his orthodox medical training he had the rare good fortune to be taught by someone who had also investigated other systems of medicine and encouraged him to keep an open mind. That advice was to save his life. After sixteen years of busy medical practice he fell seriously ill, proving, as he freely admitted later, that he knew no more about the causes of illness than anyone else! At forty years old, weighing sixteen stone (224 pounds), he was at death's door with high blood pressure, serious kidney disease and a dilated heart.

Mentally, however, he was still very much alive, and during the long nights spent fighting for breath he decided to give nature a chance. He knew that the human body is perfectly capable of healing itself if we just give it the raw material to do the job, and take away everything that hinders its work. So in came the raw material—fresh meat and vegetables, whole grains and plenty of fresh fruit and salad—and out went processed foods like sugar and white flour because they obstruct healing.

Three months later, and three stone (42 pounds) lighter, he was well on the way to recovery, much to everybody's astonishment including his own. Within a year he was fitter and stronger than ever before. Dr Hay was a medical man, yet he almost lost his life because initially he failed to see the link between diet and disease. He saw it before it was too late. Few people do.

This is a food combining diet

Although the idea of food combining is centuries old, Dr Hay did not come across it until well after his recovery. No natural whole food is cut out, foods are just served in different combinations. Concentrated proteins like meat and eggs are served with vegetables at a protein-based meal. Concentrated starches like potatoes and bread are taken at a separate vegetarian meal.

This makes digestion much easier, releases a lot more energy, and promotes healing and repair throughout the body. The range of benefits is huge and different for everybody. Long experience of natural medicine taught Dr Hay that, first and foremost, 'all disease is one thing, subject to the same rules and requiring the same treatment. It is caused by the wrong feeding every day of our lives.'

WHAT CAN I EXPECT FROM THE HAY DIET?

- Firmer flesh, firmer breasts, and softer, smoother skin.
- Thinning hair thickens, nails grow longer and stronger.
- Cellulite improves.
- PMT and menopausal symptoms are naturally relieved.
- Minor ailments clear up, saving on prescriptions and medicines.
- It strengthens resistance to candida and chronic virus infections.
- It reduces cravings and addictive tendencies.
- Wounds and ulcers heal very much faster.
- It speeds recovery from illness, even heart attacks and cancer.
- It slows down ageing and relieves much of its discomfort.
- It enhances medical treatment and natural therapies.
- Doing something constructive about the way you feel gives you a powerful boost psychologically.

Lose weight and *gain* energy

This is also a safe and sensible way to slim. You can eat as much as you need, provided you keep it natural, and snack often yet still lose weight surprisingly fast. Many of our celebrities and entertainers rely on the Hay diet to keep them fit and looking good.

THE HAY DIET IS POWERFUL

and the results can be surprisingly quick.

Here are some glimpses of what can be done

I've been on the Hay diet a month now, and I feel great. I'm ready to get up in the mornings and I'm still full of energy at the weekend. I would always put things off because I was tired. I woke up tired and I was yawning all the morning, but it never happens to me now, everything gets done. What you get out of yourself is what you put in, I'm convinced of that.

It looks as if I've found a way I can be really well at last. I've been so tired, especially that first hour in the morning. I felt jangled inside, I had pains all over my body. I was having to go to bed at half-past eight every night. I really felt I'd have to give up work and take to my bed. Well, after eight days on the Hay diet I couldn't believe how well I felt. My body feels at peace with itself now, and I even get little bursts of energy. I'm expecting great things!

My nose dripped all day from the moment I got up. It's been going on a long time but for the last four months it's been much worse. Well, it went away after just three days and I could hardly believe it!

I always felt food was important, but I never realised just how important until now. If I had consciously tried to make myself ill I couldn't have made a better job of it!

FAREWELL TO ARTHRITIS

Shirley's knees were very painful: she could not stand for long and she could not manage the stairs any more. But after three weeks' hard work on the Hay diet she was going up three flights of stairs at a time! And she celebrated of course—with a shopping spree.

IRRITABLE BOWEL

Kate was miserable. After twenty years of irritable bowel she was ready to try anything—and six weeks on the Hay diet literally transformed her. Nothing had ever helped the stomach cramps before, but as long as she keeps to her diet she is fine.

GALL BLADDER OPERATION AVOIDED

Lisa was waiting for a gall bladder operation and she looked tired out. But the pain improved so rapidly on the Hay diet that the operation proved to be unnecessary. She lost two stone (28 pounds) in three months and looks and feels a totally different person. Nowadays she can even eat fat without pain, and she stays very well so long as she keeps strictly to food combining. Lisa has also found that alcohol brings back the pain.

CHAPTER 1

The Hay Diet in a Nutshell

WHAT ARE THE RULES?

Separate *concentrated* starches from
concentrated proteins
**Cut out processed food and replace it
with natural food**
At least fifty per cent fresh fruit, vegetables and salad

FOOD COMBINING
At a starch meal
concentrated starches:
BREAD, POTATOES, RICE AND PASTA

**Salads and fresh vegetables are neutral, they go with
every meal
Fats and oils are also neutral**

At a separate protein meal
concentrated proteins:
MEAT, FISH, CHEESE AND EGGS

Food combining is only one part of the Hay diet, the first step. It is equally important to replace processed with natural food and gradually increase the amount of fresh fruit and vegetables.

Be patient, it can take a very long time to adapt

Change your eating habits slowly, at your own pace. You could, for example, concentrate on food combining at breakfast, and wait until you are comfortable with that before changing your other meals. Remember it is only the *concentrated* starches which have to be separated from *concentrated* proteins. And the occasional treat will do no harm unless you are very unwell.

HOW LONG BETWEEN A STARCH MEAL AND A PROTEIN MEAL?
Ideally wait three to four hours
Protein takes two to four hours to digest
Starch is digested mainly during the first 30–45 minutes

Snack as often as you like

- Snack on something neutral between meals if necessary.
- Near to a protein meal: snack on acid fruit.
- Near to a starch meal: snack on the sweetest fruits.

If you suffer from low blood sugar you may need to eat two-hourly.

NEUTRAL FOODS
Salads
Vegetables except potatoes
Fats and oils

* * *

Raisins, nuts and seeds
in small quantities only
Neutral foods go with both starch and protein meals

If you are still eating your usual amount of sugar, chocolate, biscuits and other processed foods then you are not fully on the Hay diet, you are just food combining. Many people can control their weight to some extent with food combining alone, but for faster weight loss and to keep really well food must be whole, it must be natural.

HOW DOES FOOD COMBINING WORK?

The theory is that concentrated starch and concentrated protein have opposite digestive requirements, so if you eat them together neither gets digested properly. Protein is digested in acid, but starch needs alkaline conditions for digestion, so they are best eaten separately.

While the body is struggling to digest incompatible mixtures of food, it often malfunctions in many other ways. Once the workload on the digestive system is reduced, the body soon gets to work putting everything else right, often in a surprising way.

When do I get results?

Minor problems can respond within days, especially digestive troubles. Long-standing problems like arthritis and asthma obviously take longer. People who benefit from food combining usually find the symptoms come back if they let it slip.

WHAT ABOUT FRUIT?

The sweeter fruits go with a starch meal: bananas, figs, dates, sweet grapes and sweet pears.

Sugar accompanies starch meals because sugar and starch both require alkaline conditions for digestion. The idea is to gradually remove refined sugar and all sweetened foods from the diet. You may be surprised to know that we do not actually need refined sugar at all: we can get all the sugar we need from fresh fruit.

With a protein meal: all the other fruits because both protein and acid fruits are digested in stomach acid.

ACID AND ALKALINE

This refers to the effect of these foods on the body once they have been digested. and absorbed. Concentrated starches like grains, and especially concentrated proteins like meat, are acid-forming in the body; they produce acid waste which is toxic in excess, so they should be taken in moderation.

- Normal body processes also produce a certain amount of acid waste.
- Processed foods are acid-forming too, and produce an unnatural amount of acid waste.
- We need plenty of alkali-forming foods to counteract the acidity.
- There is no need to separate acid and alkaline foods, they mix quite happily together.

FOR ALKALINE MEALS

Alkali-forming foods:
Fresh fruit and salad
Jacket potatoes, millet
Vegetables cooked and raw
Natural yoghurt

* * *

Nuts and seeds
in small amounts

Alkaline meals are based on fresh fruit and salad
ALKALI-FORMING FOODS SHOULD MAKE UP
50–75% OF THE HAY DIET

Why worry about which foods are acid-forming and which are alkaline?

Man developed on a diet of predominantly alkali-forming foods, mainly fresh plant foods and fruit, plus a few root vegetables and a little meat—that is our natural diet. But the balance of today's diet has gradually changed over to acid, mainly because we eat so much processed food, and so little fresh fruit and salad. An over-acid system slows us down and leads to illness. We function best on a diet which consists of mainly alkaline food, and the Hay diet follows this same natural pattern of eating.

EVERY DAY

One starch meal * One protein meal * One alkaline meal

NEVER MISS MEALS

Can I have extra meals?

Certainly. Many people find they can reduce the time between a starch and a protein meal without ill-effects so long as they don't eat the starch and the protein together.

How much food? Remember you can eat as much as you need, provided you keep it natural.

IDEALLY, DRINK MILK BETWEEN MEALS
Milk taken with cereal or other starchy foods can sometimes cause bloating and wind. It also neutralises gastric acid and can sometimes cause digestive problems, especially if taken with meat.

THE HAY DIET FOOD COMBINING CHART Do not mix starch with protein		
—combine—	—combine—	
STARCH MEALS	NEUTRAL FOODS	PROTEIN MEALS
Potatoes	Vegetables	Meat and fish
*	*except potatoes*	*
All grains:	*	Whole eggs
bread, rice, pasta	Salads and herbs	*
*	*	Hard cheese
Dried beans, peas	Nuts and seeds	Soft cheeses
and lentils	*	*
*	Fats and oils:	All fruits
Soya milk, tofu	butter and cream	*except those on*
*		*the starch list*
Egg yolk		
*		
Bananas		
Sweet pears		
Grapes		
Dates and figs		
*		
Honey		
in small amounts		

Have at least 50 per cent fresh fruit, vegetables and salad every day

This is the essence of supernutrition, essential for efficient digestion. We seriously underestimate our need for fresh food, our vitality depends on it.

A blender drink before breakfast could prove the point
Apple, cucumber and banana blended together with water and a teaspoonful of extra virgin olive oil. It can wake you up literally within minutes.

Pulses

Pulses are dried peas, beans and lentils.

- They only contain around 8% protein when cooked, so they are not concentrated proteins as so many people believe.
- Dr. Hay put them with the starch meals, but they can be taken with protein meals too.

They do not go with alkaline meals because they are acid-forming.

CHANGE OVER TO NATURAL FOOD

OUT	IN
Sugar and sweetened foods: Biscuits, cake, ice-cream Chocolate, sweets Sweet fruit yoghurts Diet yoghurts	A little honey Fresh fruit Fresh dairy cream Natural yoghurts with fresh fruit
White rice White bread White flour White pasta White crispbreads	Natural brown rice Wholemeal bread only Wholemeal flour Wholemeal pasta Wholemeal crispbreads
Cornflakes Instant oat cereals Puffed rice or wheat Sugary breakfast cereals	Shredded wheat Natural porridge oats Sugar-free muesli Wholewheat cereals
All margarines All ordinary supermarket cooking oils	Butter only *For cooking:* Butter, dripping, olive oil
Pickles and sauces Dried soups Salted nuts Potato crisps Salted snacks	Herbs and spices Home-made soups Plain, fresh nuts Sunflower seeds Pumpkin seeds
Kippers, smoked fish	Fresh or frozen fish
Processed meats: Supermarket cold meats Pork pies Bacon and ham Corned beef Sausages and beef burgers	*Any fresh, home-cooked meat:* Sliced roast meat Chops Stewing steak Liver, kidney Poultry
Textured vegetable protein (TVP)	Soya beans Tofu (soft soya cheese)

EVERYDAY FOODS
Starch-based or Protein-based Meal?

S = Starch   P = Protein   N = Neutral
+ = Alkali-forming   – = Acid-forming

Almonds	N	+	Cherries	P	+
Apples	P	+	Chestnuts	S	–
Apricots	P	+	Chicken	P	–
Artichoke	N	+	Chickpeas	S	–
Asparagus	N	+	Chicory	N	+
Aubergine	N	+	Chinese leaves	N	+
Avocado pear	N	+	Clementines	P	+
Bamboo shoots	N	+	Cockles	P	–
Bananas	S	+	Coconut	N	–
Barley	S	–	Cod	P	–
Beans			Cornmeal (maize)	S	–
dried	S	–	Courgettes (zucchini)	N	+
fresh	N	+	Crab	P	–
Beanshoots	N	+	Cream	N	N
Beef	P	–	Cress	N	+
Beetroot	N	+	Cucumber	N	+
Blackberries	P	+	Dates	S	+
Blackcurrants	P	+	Duck	P	–
Bran	N	–	Eggs, whole	P	–
Brazil nuts	N	+	yolk only	N	–
Bread	S	–	Endive	N	+
Broad beans	N	+	Figs	S	+
Broccoli	N	+	Fish	P	–
Cabbage	N	+	Garlic	N	+
Carrots	N	+	Gooseberries	P	+
Cashew nuts	N	–	Grapefruit	P	+
Cauliflower	N	+	Grapes		
Celeriac	N	+	extra sweet	S	+
Celery	N	+	sharper taste	P	+
Cheese			Hazelnuts	N	+
cottage-type	P	–	Kale	N	+
cream cheese	N	N	Kohlrabi	N	+
crumbly cheese	P	–	Kiwi fruit	P	+
hard cheese	P	–	Leeks	N	+

Lemon	P	+	Plums	P	−
Lentils	S	−	Pomegranate	P	+
Lettuce	N	+	Potato		
Limes	P	+	jacket	S	+
Linseeds	N	+	peeled	S	−
Loganberries	P	+	Prawns	P	+
Lychees	P	+	Prunes	P	−
Mango	P	+	Pumpkin seeds	N	+
Marrow	N	+	Quinoa grain	S	−
Melon (eat alone)		+	Radishes	N	+
Millet	S	+	Raisins	N	+
Mushrooms	N	+	Raspberries	P	+
Nectarine	P	+	Rhubarb	P	−
Oats	S	−	Rice, brown	S	−
oat bran	N	−	Runner beans	N	+
Okra	N	+	Rye	S	−
Olives	N	+	Satsumas	P	+
Onions	N	+	Sesame seeds	N	+
Oranges	P	+	Spinach	N	+
Papaya	P	+	Sprouted beans	N	+
Parsnips	N	+	Sprouted seeds	N	+
Passion fruit	P	+	Strawberries	P	+
Peaches	P	+	Sultanas	N	+
Peanuts (pulses)	S	−	Sunflower seeds	N	+
Pears			Swede	N	+
green	P	+	Sweetcorn	N	+
soft yellow	S	+	Sweet potato	S	+.
Peas			Tofu	S	−
fresh	N	+	Tomatoes		
dried	S	−	fresh	N	+
Pecan nuts	N	−	cooked, tinned	P	−
Peppers	N	+	Turnip	N	+
Pine nuts	N	+	Walnuts	N	−
Pineapple	P	+	Watercress	N	+
Pistachios	N	−	Yams	S	+
Plantain	S	+	Yoghurt, natural	P	+

FOOD COMBINING

Here are some practical tips to get you started.

Protein-based meals

These are usually no problem—you just eat meat or fish with vegetables as usual but without the potatoes, rice or bread. If you miss the potatoes you can serve extra vegetables.

Natural desserts
Fresh fruit with or without natural yoghurt.
Fromage frais or cottage cheese with fruit.
Dried fruit.
Egg custard.

Starch-based meals

These are vegetarian meals, without dairy products or eggs.

Starch breakfasts
Porridge or muesli with soya milk.
Wholewheat cereals and soya milk.
Toast and butter.
Grilled tomatoes or mushrooms on toast.
Vegetarian sandwiches.
Sliced banana and nuts, dates or raisins.

Starch main meals
Hearty vegetable soup and wholemeal roll.
Pitta bread filled with salad.
Jacket potato and salad.
Jacket potato and beans.
Vegetable stews and casseroles.
Rice, pasta or millet and vegetables with vegetarian sauce.
Nut roast with vegetables.

Desserts
Banana with nuts or raisins.
Dates or figs, fresh or dried.
Rice pudding made with soya milk.
Rice with raisins and banana.
Sweet grapes or sweet pear.

Alkaline meals

Vegetable soups.
Jacket potato and salad.
Fresh fruit with or without natural yoghurt.
Salad of all kinds with nuts.
Vegetable casserole, ratatouille.

Millet is the only alkali-forming grain, and a tasty alternative to rice. Millet flakes can also be used to make porridge and muesli.

The Hay Diet Made Easy, my first book, fully explains the Hay diet. It contains lists of meal ideas, ready combined for starch, protein and alkaline meals, plus plenty of menus and help with preparing natural food.

CHAPTER 2

Intelligent Weight Control

Diets don't work unless you find out why you are overweight, then deal with the underlying causes—the answers are not the same for everyone. The Hay diet is a good place to start because it takes care of most of the causes of overweight listed below. Most people find that losing weight on the Hay diet is effortless, and they feel so much better into the bargain. If you diet to slim, your health improves, and if you diet for health reasons, you lose weight if you need to. You need never be hungry, and you can literally eat yourself slim.

DOES DIETING MAKE YOU FEEL ILL?

- Sinking feelings.
- Constant hunger, never satisfied.
- A swimming head if you go without food.
- Irritable, nervous or shaky feelings before meals.
- Bingeing and compulsive eating.
- Waking at night to eat.
- Abdominal distension, especially after meals.
- Sudden tiredness and drowsiness after meals.
- Feeling ill if a meal is late.
- Craving certain foods, especially sugar.
- Digestive problems, stomach aches.
- Feeling ill with tiredness.
- Constipation.

Much of this is due to low blood sugar
YOU CAN EXPERIENCE CONSIDERABLE
RELIEF IN A SHORT TIME

Low blood sugar is very much a slimmer's problem

This is why many of us have such trouble keeping to a diet, and this is what can make us feel so tired and depressed. If you are in this position, learning to control your blood sugar could transform your life. It is fully explained in chapter 4.

WHAT ELSE CAUSES OVERWEIGHT?

Badly combined meals
Toxic overload:
Additves and preservatives
Too much processed food
Too much concentrated food
Overeating
Mercury toxicity

Fluid retention due to:
Too much salt and sugar
Lack of concentrated protein foods
Wheat intolerance
Certain drugs and hormone preparations

Lack of essential fatty acids
Chronic candida
Thyroid deficiency

Food combining

Most people are very surprised indeed at how easy it can be to lose weight once their meals are properly combined, and they are astonished at the range of other benefits. Dr Hay actually recommended getting the food combining habit well established first, before changing over to natural food.

Flatten your stomach

There are usually simple answers to abdominal distension. Many people find that food combining rapidly solves the problem—they lose inches round the waist almost straight away. If it has no effect, consider candida. Also any food to which you are intolerant can cause distension.

After keeping to food combining for three weeks I really notice how uncomfortable and full I feel if I eat starch and protein together.

The bloating went down when I cut out the apple I always ate with my sandwiches.

I'm angry. I've had this awful bloating all my life, and only now do I find out it's due to dairy products.

Whenever candida flares up again I get bloated. I feel so full up I can hardly eat.

Watch your weight carefully

If you are dieting for health reasons and you are already slim, you can easily prevent unwanted weight loss using the information in the chapters that follow.

WHY CAN I NEVER LOSE WEIGHT HOWEVER LITTLE I EAT?

When the body is repeatedly starved it tends to store what little food it gets. And if you are not eating enough of the right kind of food to provide warmth and energy, nor to keep up with body repairs, you feel cold, lethargic and ill.

Serial dieting makes you fat

Repeated short-term low calorie diets progressively slow our metabolic rate. After every diet followed by a binge, we burn food more slowly than before we started and from that time onwards we gain weight on less food. Restricted diets for food intolerance and candida can obviously have a similar effect, so make absolutely sure you get enough to eat.

Deprivation dieting can damage your health

The danger is that once our metabolism has been slowed down it can be difficult or impossible to reverse the process. Every low calorie diet not only leaves us heavier than we were before we started, it also throws our hormones out of balance and robs us of our vitality. Many people feel they have never been the same since a bout of crash-dieting, especially after childbirth or when they were unwell.

Never starve yourself—you can snack often and still lose weight

Frequent snacks of natural food are actually the best way to slim—you have to try it to believe it! Eating little and often on the Hay diet will kick-start your metabolism and keep you feeling well. These nutrition-packed meals speed up body processes, increase energy and burn off the fat.

Slim faster on regular meals

- No need to be hungry: snack as often as you need to so long as you keep it natural.
- Natural food accelerates weight loss, being less concentrated and therefore lower in calories.
- Sugar and salt are automatically restricted, reducing fluid retention.

36

- As the toxins stored in cellulite are released, the fat disappears too.
- Fifty per cent fresh fruit and salad provides the vitamins and minerals required to shift the fat.
- Regular meals and blood sugar control help the hormone system to recover its balance.

It works!

I hardly ever ate, I just had coffee all day, and a sandwich, yet I never ever lost weight. It didn't make sense. But now I'm on the Hay diet with regular meals I've lost five stone (70 pounds), and I've never felt better!

I was losing weight fine on regular meals, then went back onto a low-calorie diet to speed things up but the weight loss stopped; I was at a standstill again! You live and learn!

FOOD CRAVINGS

Unnatural food = unnatural hunger

Hunger is just the body's search for nutrients. You can eat a whole packet of biscuits and still crave more, you still feel something is missing—and it is! These cravings are deceptive. Your body is crying out, not for another biscuit but for all the vitamins and minerals which have been processed out of it. You can experience natural hunger and a much more contented stomach on natural food. It astonishes most people how fast such cravings can disappear.

ARE YOU A CHOCOHOLIC?

Amazingly, many people have no trouble at all giving it up on the Hay diet with blood sugar control.

Hunger and cravings, especially for sugar, happen when blood sugar levels fall below normal. But refined sugar is not the answer because it is absorbed too fast and floods the system. Insulin then removes the excess from the bloodstream, rapidly converts it to fat, and deposits it on hips, thighs—anywhere!

CHRONIC CANDIDA

Slimmers who find it impossible to give up sugar despite the Hay diet and blood sugar control, may also be suffering from candida. The cravings it can create for sugar, bread and alcohol create severe weight problems for many people—see chapter 7.

WHEAT INTOLERANCE AND COMPULSIVE EATING

It is possible to crave any food if you are allergic to it, but wheat is the most common cause of abdominal discontent, and a major unrecognised contributor to overweight. I was always hungry, with a baffling inner tension which constantly drove me to look for food. I could never get enough to eat and I could never start the day without my Weetabix. When I cut wheat out altogether the withdrawal symptoms were awful—I felt so hungry I could have eaten the table and the chair. I should have reduced it more gradually. Even now, after years without it, if I start eating bread again I find I just can't stop eating all day. All the gluten grains (wheat, rye, barley and oats) make me incredibly depressed into the bargain, so I never touch them now.

Wheat takes a long time to leave the system
If you cut it out it may be anything up to three weeks before you feel better.

ARE YOU ZINC DEFICIENT?

Cravings for food in general are sometimes due to zinc deficiency (see p. 204).

ARE YOU EATING THE WRONG KIND OF FAT?

Overweight people are usually lacking in the essential fatty acids found in extra virgin olive oil, nuts, seeds, avocado pears and fresh oily fish. Everybody needs them in moderation. Low fat diets which forbid these essential fats and oils are a health hazard—see chapter 13.

Fat delays emptying of the stomach

A meal which contains fat is therefore more sustaining. Natural, unrefined vegetable oils are essential to the proper absorption of many nutrients. The Hay diet, combined with one or two tablespoons of extra virgin olive oil a day, produces firmer flesh which is more evenly distributed.

Toxic overload creates cellulite, which is toxic fat

Cellulite is the ugly dimpled fat which gets packed solid on thighs and buttocks and is so difficult to shed. Many pesticides, additives and preservatives, especially those which are used to prevent fats and oils from going rancid, are fat soluble. The liver destroys many of these harmful substances, but if we take them to excess they are often stored out of harm's way in body fat.

Mercury is also stored in fat!

Mercury, too, adds to the toxic load, and the more amalgam fillings you have the worse it is. As you detoxify, the fat can melt away. Read the case history on p. 229.

NATURAL FOOD IS LIGHTER, LESS CONCENTRATED

We tend to become overweight if we eat too much concentrated, processed food. Fresh fruit and vegetables contain more water and provide more bulk. They satisfy on fewer calories, and the fibre they contain speeds the passage of food through the body and eases constipation.

SUGAR AND SALT OVERSTIMULATE THE APPETITE

They trick us into eating more than we need, as food manufacturers are very well aware!

OVEREATING MAKES MORE WASTE FOR THE BODY TO DISPOSE OF

It overworks the system and can be tiring. Excess starch and protein, too, can be turned into fat.

ARE YOU A PROBLEM SLIMMER?

Evening primrose oil can sometimes help

It has been known to activate the special brown fat which lies at the back of the neck and along the spine. When it is working normally, brown fat burns off excess calories as heat, otherwise they turn to fat. Evening primrose oil can only work with people who are at least ten per cent over their ideal body weight, and then usually only with those who are severely overweight, with a strong family history of obesity. There is more information in *Evening Primrose Oil* by Judy Graham.

Thyroid deficiency

An underactive thyroid gland can lead to mental and physical sluggishness and overweight. A blood test for thyroid deficiency can be obtained from your GP.

FLUID RETENTION

It is well known that salt can cause fluid retention, but refined sugar is so highly concentrated that it too can have this effect. Remember that sugar and salt are automatically reduced on the Hay diet. A large weight loss in a short time is usually due to fluid loss; losing fat takes time and patience.

Drink plenty of water

The body dilutes toxins in water, sometimes leading to fluid retention. But you still need at least a litre of water a day; it provides the body with a clean supply of water and helps to flush out the toxins. Cellulite also contains water.

Lack of protein can also cause fluid retention

Everyone needs concentrated protein every day, so if you are overweight and your diet contains little or no meat, eggs, cheese or fish, this could be part of the answer.

ALLERGIES CAN MAKE YOU FAT

Allergic fluid retention is another common reason for over-weight, and once you identify and remove the offending food the weight loss can be rapid. Again, people with severe weight problems are often intolerant of wheat and/or dairy products, especially cheese and milk chocolate, which they may consume in large amounts.

Wheat was Sally's problem

I've struggled to keep my weight down for years, ever since my early teens. Then a homoeopath suggested I cut out wheat and over the next nine months I lost two and a half stone (35 pounds) without really trying. I could hardly believe it.
There is more information in chapter 9.

AVOID HIGH PROTEIN DIETS WHICH ARE LOW IN STARCH

If our diet is high in animal protein but low in starch, we have to break down the protein for fuel, and that creates an unnatural amount of toxic debris, more than some of us can handle. Knowing nothing of the long-term dangers, we may not associate any health problems we may have with our high protein intake.

In the long term a high protein diet can contribute to:

- Fatigue, gum disease, skin problems.
- Gout, arthritis, osteoporosis.
- Degenerative disease including cancer.
- Constipation through lack of fibre; it can sometimes be severe, causing acute abdominal pain.

The Hay diet is safer by far.

DRUGS AND HORMONES CAN PUT ON WEIGHT

If you have suddenly gained a lot of weight, look back to see if you made changes in your life around the time it began. Certain drugs and hormone preparations can cause generalised fluid retention, leading to massive weight gain in some people. Also, the toxins they produce are often stored out of harm's way in fat especially manufactured for that purpose.

Madeleine's story

Madeleine's problems began with the contraceptive pill, and they grew worse on hormone treatment. She gained seven stone (98 pounds) and her hair got very thin. Like most people of her size she was a hopeless chocoholic, but only before her periods; she did not touch it at other times. She took Glanolin and worked amazingly hard on the Hay diet and blood sugar control. By the end of a month she had lost twenty pounds and all the bloating was gone. Her PMT was down from ten days to two, and she had even managed to give up her chocolate.

She loved cheese, too, but found that her chest and sinus problems improved greatly without dairy products. And best of all, her hair was beginning to grow again all round the hairline —she was thrilled. Before the Hay diet she had been doing five miles a day on her exercise bike, but now she was losing weight without it. By the end of four months she had lost three stone (42 pounds), but alas, she slackened off over Christmas. The PMT came back with a vengeance, and her period was agony. A great learning experience!

NOTE: Glanolin is blackcurrant seed oil, sometimes used instead of Evening Primrose Oil.

A miracle?

Tracey came in search of a miracle. Her diet was chaotic; she often missed breakfast and felt faint by lunchtime, but she had a good meal every evening. She had a cola drink every day and she was a smoker, too. She woke up tired and found it difficult to get up. She had crying spells, she was depressed and constantly stressed. Some days she felt well, at other times she felt she was going to pieces. She always had PMT with migraine and at this time of the month she suffered uncontrollable cravings for bread and sweet things. She would binge on chocolate until she felt sick, so she was very overweight. Frightening dizzy spells sent her rushing to the doctor in a panic two or three times a week. The doctor felt they were due to low blood sugar but he could not help.

Over the next month she cut out sugar and stimulants, and she ate natural food every two hours on the Hay diet. She also took high dose multivitamin tablets and evening primrose oil.

I've lost six pounds and I've never been able to lose weight before. I stuck to the Hay diet and I felt great until I had mint sauce. It was loaded with sugar and I didn't know. I had the most terrible reaction. My colour drained away, I felt sick and dizzy, my whole body felt on fire. I went rushing to the GP again and he said, 'Your blood pressure is so low I don't know how you're managing to stand up, and your blood sugar level is at rock bottom.' I just couldn't get up next morning, it took me four days to get over it.

FOUR MONTHS LATER
I've come out of that bad patch now, and I've never had another asthma attack since I've been on the Hay diet. I never have sugar or coffee and I feel terrific. I only go to the GP surgery once a month now to get my weight checked, and they can hardly believe the difference in me. It's like a new life.

* * *

WOULD YOU LIKE TO PUT ON WEIGHT?

It can actually sometimes be more of a problem to gain weight than to lose it; some of us have to keep a very strict eye on our weight because we lose it so easily. But on the Hay diet you can put on plenty of firm flesh, often in quite a short time, without resorting to sugar. The secret, I have found, is to take plenty of the natural unrefined oils, especially extra virgin olive oil, plus avocado pears and the other foods naturally rich in essential fats. This is the only thing that worked for me, after many years of searching for answers.

Weight gain depends on having enough of the right kind of fat in the diet

Enzymes break down food ready for absorption, and a quarter of all our enzyme systems depend on fats: they are essential to almost every bodily function. And remember that the absorption of fat-soluble vitamins A and E from the intestine also depends on having adequate fats and oils. So very gradually increase your intake of natural oils until your weight begins to creep upwards.

You may need up to two or three ounces of oil spread over the day:

- You can use any of the natural unrefined oils from the health food shop—sunflower, safflower, light sesame, corn oil, or extra virgin olive oil. Vary the oils, and take them with cooked vegetables or salad. The antioxidant vitamins in the salad prevent the oil from turning rancid in the body.
- Natural vitamin E—D alpha tocopherol—in oil capsules, also prevents rancidity.
- Whole grains combined with extra virgin olive oil are a body-building combination.
- When you have gained enough weight you can gradually reduce the oils to a level which keeps your weight steady.

Don't worry about taking so much oil. Remember that we are already in the habit of consuming large amounts of fat hidden in cakes, biscuits and confectionery.

BUT BE CAREFUL TO AVOID NAUSEA!
Increase the oil very gradually indeed, and always incorporate it into other foods. There is more information in chapter 13.

CAUTION: Sudden unexplained loss of weight needs to be investigated by a doctor.

MORE SUGGESTIONS FOR PUTTING ON WEIGHT

Food combining helps to normalise weight
Interestingly, it can also help you to gain weight because food is better absorbed.

Make sure you get enough to eat over the day
If we are to build flesh, not flab, food must be natural, and in order to gain weight there must be nutrients to spare. If eating tires you out or if you have trouble digesting larger meals, you may need to eat little and often so as not to overload the system.

Make sure you get enough concentrated foods
Especially you need whole grains and potatoes. Concentrated proteins like meat help to build muscle, and remember that protein is easier to digest if you take it with plenty of salad.

Consider food intolerance
You may find that you are intolerant of certain foods, and that by identifying the culprits and removing them from the diet you can then put on weight. Dairy products and wheat are common offenders.

Mercury can reduce the appetite and impair digestion
I have been able to eat much more food and digest it much more easily since having my amalgam fillings removed. That, too, has helped me to gain weight.

COELIAC DISEASE

This condition is becoming more widespread, and many cases still go undiagnosed even though it is recognised by the medical profession. It is an intolerance to gluten, the protein part of wheat, rye, barley and oats, which prevents food from being properly absorbed. It is very common in children, too.

Consider coeliac disease if:
- You are painfully thin despite a good appetite.
- You have loose stools.
- You have to rush to the toilet two or three times a day.

- You have mysterious diarrhoea which does not respond to treatment.

You could try gradually cutting out wheat, rye, barley and oats, and replacing them with potatoes and plenty of the gluten-free grains, to see if it makes any difference.

WHAT ARE THE GLUTEN-FREE GRAINS?
Rice, millet, buckwheat and quinoa. They all cook as for rice, although cooking times vary.

If it clears up when you exclude gluten:
You can then be tested for coeliac disease at the local hospital, and in Britain gluten-free bread is free of charge on medical prescription.

GLUTEN-FREE PRODUCTS CAN BE VERY EXPENSIVE

- Many health food shops sell gluten-free products.
- You can order gluten-free bread and flour through any chemist in the UK without a medical prescription.

The Coeliac Society produces a comprehensive food list, a 166-page booklet, updated annually, listing every conceivable gluten-free manufactured product on sale in Britain, including gluten-free pasta and breads. The address of the Coeliac Society will be found in Useful Addresses.

You may prefer to eat naturally
Remember that commercial gluten-free products are mostly made from refined flour and are usually highly processed. Some people may prefer to go without bread and baked goods altogether, relying on potatoes and rice, plus the other gluten-free grains, if you can tolerate them.

Intolerance to whole wheat and other grains

Most of the gluten-free flours contain wheat starch, so gluten-free diets do not help everyone. Many other people, myself included, cannot take wheat, rye, barley or oats in any form, and some have problems with the gluten-free grains too. There is more information in chapter 9.

JOHN'S STORY

John had always been far too thin, even as a child, despite a very good appetite. And he had always had to rush to the toilet two or three times a day. In middle age he began to find that an increasing number of ordinary foods gave him diarrhoea, especially fruits. Then came a really severe attack of diarrhoea which doctors could not stop. In desperation he cut out wheat, rye and oats (bread, cakes and biscuits, rye crispbreads and porridge) and it cleared up in no time, so the doctor sent him to the hospital, where tests confirmed that he had coeliac disease. He gained weight fast on a gluten-free diet, for the first time ever, and now can tolerate all the other foods that were upsetting him. But now alas, he has a new problem, he has to struggle to keep his weight down!

NOTE: The information given above is not meant to be a complete guide to coeliac disease.

CHAPTER 3

How Well Do You Want to Be?

You only have to look at the soaring cost of the health services and the rising tide of illness to know that we must be missing something which affects absolutely everybody, something with slow, insidious effects. We tend to assume that the average diet is healthy, however unhealthy we may be. We grow up with the impression that food has very little to do with the way we feel from day to day, but the evidence suggests otherwise.

Cancer and heart disease were far less common in the early part of the twentieth century, when food was more natural. Food-processing is having a devastating effect on our lives; vital ingredients are going missing, and many of us are becoming mysteriously tired and run-down as a result. The Hay diet, however, being completely natural, releases all the energy tied up by processed food so that we can use it for other things. Most people are astonished at how much better they feel and very soon realise that our choice of food matters much more than we realise.

We are right to be concerned about genetically modified foods, but familiar everyday foods whose safety we have always taken for granted, highly processed foods like sugar, white flour and highly processed fats, are equally unnatural to the body. Good health is good function, when body and mind are operating at peak performance, but average health is all we can expect on today's diet. From early childhood body and mind begin to malfunction in many different ways.

THIS IS AVERAGE HEALTH!

Headaches	Aches and pains
Frequent infections	Period pains
Low blood sugar	Mental tiredness
Fatigue, low energy	Irritability
Poor concentration	Pale complexion
Constipation	Greasy hair
Skin problems	Emotional problems
Occasional depression	Feeling unwell at times
Body odour	Digestive problems
Joint pains	Stomach aches
Nervous problems	Mood swings

THERE IS NO NEED TO LIVE LIKE THIS

What does average health mean?

It means being well enough to work or to study, and over the years it frequently means stoically accepting an increasing number of nervous problems and minor ailments of all kinds. But this is where degeneration begins; these are the early-warning signs of more serious illness.

BUT EVERYONE HAS A HEALTH PROBLEM
OF SOME KIND, DON'T THEY?
Most people with problems like these would nevertheless consider themselves fit because they have nothing seriously wrong—yet. But there is absolutely no need to live like this. Such problems are usually reversible, and easy to deal with ourselves once we know more about food.

WHY WAIT FOR SOMETHING SERIOUS TO HAPPEN?
Being equally unaware of the importance of natural foods, many doctors, too, 'wait for something to happen'—to find evidence of disease or damage—and we follow their lead. We conscientiously maintain our cars but neglect our most precious asset, ignoring the needs of our own body until our health breaks down.

THERE IS A SERIOUS GAP IN OUR EDUCATION
We naively expect our body to work properly without any help or understanding from us. We have little idea of its needs, and we know precious little about how to help ourselves when we are ill. Most of us still firmly believe that the average diet contains enough vitamins and minerals to keep us fit, and that diet does not play a significant part in illness, but the reality is that today's diet contains enough nutrients to prevent the serious

---

THIS IS POSITIVE HEALTH—PEAK PERFORMANCE

Muscular strength	A strong, supple body
Freedom from aches and pains	A positive feeling of well-being
Steady nerves, stable mood	Sound sleep, easy waking
Regular bowel movements	Strength and stamina
Clear thinking, creativity	Good short-term memory
Easy concentration	Positive thinking
A wide-awake, alert mind	High energy
Clear, soft, supple skin	A healthy head of hair
Confidence and self-control	Steady weight, firm flesh
Kindliness and good humour	Interest and enthusiasm

THIS IS OUR NATURAL STATE

---

malnutrition that leads to scurvy and rickets, but is not nearly good enough to keep us positively well.

People living in rural communities where food is plentiful and has always been completely natural, normally have a strikingly good physique and handsome posture. Their energy is boundless and they radiate good humour. But a trouble-free body and mind like this seldom come naturally on today's diet. It requires supernutrition, it requires commitment. There is a huge gap between what we are and what we could be, physically, emotionally and intellectually.

Few of us today have ever lived entirely without processed food. People who travel to faraway places where food is natural, where they cannot obtain their usual treats, miss them terribly at first but come back feeling fantastic, thoroughly convinced that we really are what we eat. This is the kind of experience anyone can have on the Hay diet.

YOU MAY NEED TO TAKE EXTRA CARE OF YOURSELF

Nature works hard to restore normal function to every organ in the body, but if you have been ill for a very long time, and especially if you have taken powerful medication over a long period, you may have to settle for less. If you are seriously below par mentally and physically, you will need a period of intensive care. Like a house that has fallen into disrepair over many years, your body will require a lot of attention over a long time. Nevertheless, the quality of your life could improve beyond measure, and the improvement continues indefinitely.

One in ten of us needs supernutrition
ALL THE TIME!
THE HAY DIET IS A HIGH-PERFORMANCE DIET
It could give you a new lease of life

Some of us have to be very careful indeed what we eat, every day of our lives. Experts estimate that as many as one in ten of us can only ever function normally—physically, socially and intellectually—on a well-balanced natural diet, without processed food as far as possible, and a number of us find we are intolerant of some of the natural foods, too. So if you are struggling along on a 'normal' diet, the information in this book could change your life.

Is your diet your biggest obstacle?

Too many of us, talented and potentially very able people, are under-achievers. We struggle through life, never dreaming that all that holds us back is unsuitable food. An inappropriate diet can even rob us of a livelihood. Yet with supernutrition, beginning with the Hay diet, many such people are transformed, and can make their hopes and dreams a reality.

THESE ARE THE DANGER FOODS

Refined carbohydrates:
Sugar, chocolate, biscuits, cakes, ice-cream
All other sweetened foods
Alcohol and soft drinks, especially cola
White flour, white bread, white rice and white pasta

Processed meats, fats and fried food:
Sausages, spam, ham
Margarines and cooking oils
Salted snacks, potato crisps

Highly processed foods are very much second rate from the body's point of view. Too many convenience foods and too little fresh food, combined with a busy, stressful life, continually run down our stocks of vitamins and the many other vital nutrients, so unless we put back what we are taking out, we are heading for trouble. People whose health breaks down in a serious way, with cancer or mental illness, with M.E. or a heart attack, can often look back and see exactly what led to their illness.

SUGAR AND ALL SWEETENED FOODS

drain us of:
Calcium, chromium, manganese and zinc
Vitamins A, B, C and E

Tea, coffee, alcohol
and highly processed foods
have a similar effect

They can upset our hormone balance too
THEY ARE A MAJOR CAUSE OF MALNUTRITION

DIET BEFORE VITAMIN PILLS!
Many of us carry on eating carelessly, believing that if we take a daily vitamin and mineral supplement all will be well, but vitamin tablets can never fully compensate for the deficiencies created by junk food. The first essential is a natural diet.

BUT WHY CAN SOME PEOPLE APPARENTLY EAT AND
DRINK WHATEVER THEY LIKE?
Undoubtedly some of us inherit a more efficient liver than others, one which detoxifies the system more effectively. Like the miner's canary, susceptible people suffer first, but the others will run into trouble eventually if they continue their unhealthy lifestyle.

Internal pollution

Our strength and resistance to illness largely depend on being able to rid ourselves fast of the acid waste produced by body cells each day; it happens automatically on an all-natural diet because natural food leaves very little waste. But junk food produces more debris than we can handle—'internal filth' was Dr Hay's view of it.

CLEAR YOUR COMPLEXION
A greyish, muddy complexion is further evidence of toxic acid build-up. You can often see it in heavy smokers and in people who are very run down and ill, but it gradually clears up on the Hay diet. As explained in chapter 1, at least 50 per cent fresh fruit and salad is essential to keep the system clean.

————*WHAT ELSE ADDS TO THE TOXIC LOAD?*————

- Additives, preservatives, pesticides.
- Foods to which we are intolerant are also toxic to us.
- Drugs of all kinds can produce toxic side-effects.
- Mercury toxicity from amalgam dental fillings.
- Tobacco and too much alcohol.
- Stress slows down toxin elimination.

Remember the healing principle:
Give the body the tools for the job and take away everything that hinders its work.

What about organic food?

By all means eat organically if you can afford it, you will feel better for it; but you can still recover without it. Home-grown vegetables are a good idea.

THE SACCHARINE DISEASE

This is a master disease covering the many conditions related to the consumption of sugar and white flour—remember that the body turns starch to sugar. It has nothing to do with artificial sweeteners. The connection was made by the late Surgeon Captain T.L. Cleave of the Royal Navy, a pioneer researcher whose work is still not being taken seriously. He wrote *The Saccharine Disease* which clearly explains how it all happens.

THIS IS THE SACCHARINE DISEASE
(Saccharine rhymes with 'Rhine')

Constipation	Tooth decay, gum disease
Diverticulitis	Gallstones
Varicose veins	Stomach ulcers
Diabetes	Appendicitis
Coronary thrombosis	Bowel cancer

**People who cannot obtain sugar and white flour
and who live entirely on natural food
seldom suffer these problems**

Beware hidden sugar

Many of us no longer add sugar to food and drinks at home, so most of the sugar we now consume is hidden in the ready-made cakes, biscuits, ice-cream and the other sugary foods we buy from supermarkets. And because sugar is also added to many savoury foods nowadays, we may not realise just how much sugar we are actually having.

A FURTHER WORD OF WARNING ABOUT SUGAR

Too much sugar, and too many sweet foods and drinks, can demineralise the bones, robbing us of calcium in particular. This is what leads to crowded teeth in so many of our children and teenagers. The late Dr Weston Price, a retired dentist, travelled the world in search of evidence of this. The photographs he took are a revelation, and can be seen in his classic work *Nutrition and Physical Degeneration*—and obviously sugar makes a major contribution to osteoporosis, too.

White bread, white flour, white rice, white pasta
Although these are less refined than sugar, they still turn to concentrated sugar in the body (see p. 88).

WHY BOTHER TO CHANGE YOUR DIET?

Consider a stomach problem, for example:
Indigestion is a signal to us that we are eating the wrong food, but if we misunderstand the message and just treat the symptoms with medicine:

- We have to keep on taking the medicine because the way we are eating continues to irritate our stomach.
- If an ulcer then develops, we treat that with more medicine.
- If the irritation from the wrong food persists over many years, it puts us at risk from cancer.

Cancer is a chronic illness

Much cancer is produced by long-term irritation of the tissues and by chronic poisoning of the body as a whole. A major stressful episode can be the last straw. An operation to remove the tumour can be a life-saver, but if we continue our destructive eating habits, the toxic build-up continues as before and we risk a recurrence.

NATURAL INTENSIVE CARE

There is actually a natural detoxification programme for cancer, based on organic food, devised by the late Dr Max Gerson, another medical convert to natural medicine. He saved many lives. Beata Bishop made a complete recovery from malignant melanoma using Gerson therapy and tells her remarkable story in her very readable book, *A Time to Heal*.

WHY SO MUCH FRESH FOOD?

Just as a successful organic farmer understands the laws of nature and works with it, so we have to learn more about food and the way our body works, and work with it if we are to recover naturally. Our bodies have not changed, but our diet has, drastically. Nowadays the average diet may contain little salad, fresh fruit, or vegetables, often none at all. But we are still part of nature, and we pay a heavy price if we forget it.

Fresh fruit, raw vegetables and salads are natural convenience foods

Just increase them gradually.

Here are some suggestions to get you started:

- Make fresh fruit and fruit juice part of your breakfast.
- Substitute PURE diluted fruit juice for soft drinks.
- Substitute fresh fruit for snack foods and sweet desserts.
- Have a good salad-based meal at least once a day.
- Place a large bowl of fresh mixed salad on the table at every meal. You could start a meal with it or fill yourself up from the salad bowl afterwards.

You will be very surprised to find that salad with a meal actually makes it far more satisfying. It reduces hunger and cravings by giving the body enough vitamins and minerals to digest food properly.

58

ARE YOU EATING LITTLE OR NO FRESH FRUIT OR SALAD?

Do you . . .
- lack vitality?
- look run-down and unfit?
- tend to be physically and mentally sluggish?
- lack motivation and concentration?
- have skin problems, especially acne?
- suffer various other minor ailments?

Are you . . .
- allergic?
- overweight?
- prone to depression and nervous problems?
- plagued by infections, especially in winter?

MORE FRESH FRUIT AND SALAD BRINGS RAPID RELIEF
The more you have, the faster and better the results.
At least 50 per cent of your diet

And don't forget the salad oil
You will soon acquire the taste for the natural unrefined oils, they are full of flavour.

- Mix extra virgin olive oil, or a blend of the other oils, with lemon juice to taste, and keep it on the table in a bottle to sprinkle over salad.

People in Europe and throughout the Middle East have always lived like this, and their cookbooks are fully of exciting salad ideas. You will soon come to enjoy shopping for it and preparing it.

Which foods should I choose?

Just eat as wide a variety as you can to ensure you get enough nutrients. Be adventurous, try new fruits and vegetables and persevere with them.

ALL THESE ARE SUPERFOODS

Red and yellow fruits and vegetables
Dark green leafy vegetables
Avocado pears
Kiwi fruits
Citrus fruits
Beetroot, beansprouts

We cannot afford to be ill. We cannot afford the time, the expense or the disruption of our routine. A good resistance to stress, allergy and infection depends on having adequate body stocks of vitamins and minerals to draw on in an emergency. Winter colds and viruses can become a thing of the past if you keep to the Hay diet.

- Living food is vital for body repairs and maintenance, and for better digestion.
- Minerals, essential oils and the fat-soluble vitamins A, D and E can all be stored in the body, but not vitamin C or the B vitamins—and they are all abundant in fresh fruit and salad.
- Although fresh fruit and salad are low in calories they are extremely high in energy because, like spark plugs, they release the energy from other foods, especially starch and fat. You soon begin to look and feel much brighter, you wake earlier and go to bed later, quite naturally.

Anyone who is ill needs supernutrition

It takes a much higher level of nutrients to restore health than to maintain it. We need vitamins and minerals in their natural state, from fresh food, for quick and easy absorption. Processed foods give the body a lot of unnecessary work, at a time when it should be concentrating all its efforts on fighting illness.

'IF YOU KILL YOUR FOOD IT WILL SURELY KILL YOU'

This observation was made by the Essene Brotherhood, who wrote the Dead Sea Scrolls, and there is a large element of truth in it. Highly processed food which keeps for an unnaturally long time is dead; the living ingredients have been removed to increase shelf life. Fresh food spoils fast, but the faster it is likely to spoil, the more biologically active it is and the more vitality we get from it.

The living enzymes in fresh fruit and salad break down food to its individual components, ready to be rebuilt as human tissue.

- Enzymes die at around 104°F (40°C) so they are killed by cooking.
- Enzymes are also vitamin-dependent and need a rich supply of vitamins to do their work—and remember that cooking destroys vitamins, too.
- Fresh fruit and salad come complete with a perfect combination of vitamins, minerals and enzymes.

BOOST YOUR IMMUNITY WITH FRESH FOOD

The immune system is like a battery: natural food recharges it with vitamins and minerals. Junk food is vitamin-deficient and runs it down.

BUT I DON'T HAVE TIME TO LOOK AFTER MYSELF LIKE THAT!

More fresh fruit and salad means less cooking, and if you persevere with the Hay diet you will find it adds more hours to your day, more than making up for any extra time spent preparing meals.

Life without highly processed food makes shopping a lot easier, too. With a minimum of packaged foods there is little need to worry about hidden additives and preservatives.

Natural food can be cheaper

- Compare the cost of natural porridge oats with a packet of cornflakes.
- Fresh fruit makes a delicious and inexpensive snack or dessert.
- You are more satisfied on less food.
- You could grow your own.

Most greengrocers and supermarkets in Britain have a bargain box containing fresh food which is slightly marked or past its sell-by date, but often still perfectly fresh.

But I have no appetite for raw food!
The vitamin and mineral supplement programme on p. 202 can sometimes help you get started.

Raw food upsets my stomach

- You could try stir-frying or steaming it lightly.
- Once you have removed processed food from the diet and are separating starch from protein, you may well find that your digestion improves and you can tolerate it better.
- Problems digesting raw food can sometimes be a feature of food intolerance, especially to wheat, and of coeliac dis-

ease. Once the offending food is removed you may find that your body copes with it better.

- A Japanese macrobiotic diet, which is another healing diet based on cooked vegetables and brown rice, may suit you better if you still find it impossible to take raw food.

FRESH FRUIT AND SALAD ARE IMMENSELY REWARDING

This is high performance fuel, you get more work done on it.

- It enhances creativity.
- It is body-building.
- It speeds natural healing.
- It promotes mental and emotional stability.

People live longer on natural food, too. It is more in tune with a more natural way of living.

More comments from the converted

I'm only eating pure natural food now. I've lost fifteen pounds and I've never felt better. Energy? I'm bursting with it, I was amazed.

Whenever I'm ill or not right I go back on the Hay diet. It clears me right out, and I can lose half a stone whenever I need to.

I had three days on painkillers at every period, I'd have to take time off work, but since I've changed my diet it hasn't happened.

We always eat properly. I'm sure that if I were to eat white bread and cakes it would have an effect on me mentally and physically. I'd try it for a week except that I've got such a demanding job—I need to be on top of things all the time.

After fresh fruit salad for breakfast I feel better literally after twenty minutes, I feel so terrific on it.

No wonder I was ill, not a single piece of fruit, no salad, no vegetables. Since I've been on the Hay diet I've experienced a minor miracle. I've lost weight and I feel marvellous.

DIET BEFORE EXERCISE

There is no need to punish yourself. You can improve your level of fitness much faster and make exercise a lot more enjoyable if you start with a high-energy, natural diet. The average person will find the Hay diet is all they need.

Never push yourself if you are unwell

Too much exercise can drain you if you do it before you are ready. As your diet improves, muscle tone improves too and your strength and stamina gradually return. But be very careful because extra strength and vitality are required for strenuous exercise. We can only benefit from it if there are sufficient reserves of nutrients available to meet the demand for energy. So any attempts to get fit will have to be backed up by sound nutrition over a considerable time beforehand if you are very debilitated, and you will also need the vitamin and mineral programme on p. 202. So listen to your body, keep within your physical limitations, and they will extend quite naturally. Gentle stretching may be all that you can manage at first.

The road to recovery

It opens up before you as your understanding grows. There is so much more you can do about the way you feel. This is simple dietary therapy, part of the traditional art of medicine. It is safe, inexpensive, and it works surprisingly fast.

IMPROVE YOUR DIGESTION WITH THE
HAY DIET

No natural food contains both *concentrated* starch and *concentrated* protein together, either starch or protein predominates, and food combining works by applying this same natural principle to our meals.

CHEW THOROUGHLY
It helps to put your spoon or your knife and fork down between mouthfuls whenever you have the time.

TAKE MORE WATER WITH IT!
Fresh fruit, vegetables and salad have a high water content and are light and easy on the digestion. Concentrated foods like meat and potatoes are heavy, containing very little water, and can be much more difficult to digest.

If you are very debilitated or have severe digestive problems: adding water to potatoes and rice can make them a lot more digestible.

- Potatoes can be liquidised to make potato soup or a sauce to pour over other vegetables.
- Rice and any of the other grains can be liquidised to make porridge.
- Cooked meat can be blended with cooked vegetables or salad to make a soup.
- Meat can be finely minced.
- Eggs can be scrambled.

Only add enough water to enable you to digest your food comfortably. We do need some concentrated food for warmth and energy and to maintain our body weight. It may mean eating little and often in order to get enough to eat. I have had to liquidise rice and potatoes myself for many years.

Meat, fish, cheese and eggs are much easier to digest if you take them with plenty of salad.

BEAT CONSTIPATION

A major cause of constipation is refined carbohydrate. Sugar, white flour, white pasta and white rice are all stripped of their fibre and can therefore clog the bowel. Incompatible mixtures of food add to the problem, as does the general lack of fresh fruit and salad in our diet. The Hay diet alone solves the problem for many people, but others may need more help.

Natural remedies for constipation

A backlog of faeces can build up despite passing regular stools, especially if a stool is only passed once every two or three days. You would feel a lot better if you could pass a stool every day, and simple measures may be all you need to achieve it.

FOOD COMBINING
Separating starch from protein often relieves constipation of long standing, because food then moves through the system faster. The natural fibre in fruit and vegetables also eases the passage of food through the bowel.

Drink plenty of fluid, one litre a day at least—water or natural drinks only.
Plenty of extra virgin olive oil can be a great help.
Corn on the cob is very high in fibre and extremely effective as a natural aperient.
Beans and peas can have a similar effect.
Linseeds or Linusit Gold which is crushed linseeds in sealed foil packets, can help constipation and provide other far-reaching health benefits.
Ground psyllium husks are a natural plant fibre which adds

bulk to the stools, so that the bowel gets a better grip on the food and moves it along faster. It absorbs water, so you need plenty of fluid with it, otherwise it can be constipating. It is more economical to buy it loose (see address on p. 240).

Oat bran is gentle. Wheat bran can sometimes be irritating and constipating.

Aperients. Most people find they work for a while, but if taken regularly they lose their effect. They may still work if used only very occasionally. Avoid straining, as it encourages haemorrhoids (piles). You could follow up an aperient with a glycerine suppository the next day.

Clear the bowel and keep it clear

This is a basic rule of internal hygiene. Long-term constipation increases the risk of bowel cancer. Many people who pass a regular stool, perhaps every other day, live with a loaded bowel, it is never really empty. Some of us eventually become so constipated that we completely lose the natural urge to pass a stool. The bowel can become so weak, so lacking in muscle tone, that it no longer has the strength to expel the faeces. If you are reasonably thin you may be able to feel a hard, lumpy, loaded bowel through your abdominal wall if you lie down. This can be a good way to check whether or not you have completely cleared it. Normal function can often be restored to the most constipated bowel if you are prepared to work at it.

CLEARING A LOADED BOWEL
If constipation has built up over several days, you will be feeling decidedly toxic and uncomfortable. A weakened bowel obviously has a better chance of working with only one day's waste to expel.

Try glycerine suppositories first
You may need them more than once a day; you will know when you are ready to pass another stool. Do not wait for the natural

urge, it may not come. Just insert the suppository when you feel that more faeces have moved lower down into the bowel.

Help nature out!

- A drink of hot water.
- A cold flannel placed on the lower back.

Lean right forward on the toilet with your hands touching the floor, and bend your knees back, to be as near as possible to the natural squatting position.

If suppositories do not work
Try an enema. Commercial enemas can be bought ready-prepared in plastic bags with a nozzle, from any chemist. They are suitable for occasional use.

MERCURY AND CONSTIPATION
Mercury vapour from dental fillings dissolves into the saliva and passes down into the gut. Removing mercury can some-times help constipation in a remarkable way, by improving the muscle tone in the bowel. It worked for me.

Colonic irrigation

This can be the answer to stubborn constipation, foul wind, and a 'dirty gut'. You will know if you have one! See page 246–249.

CHAPTER 4

Introducing Low Blood Sugar

Are you often tired and unable to think properly before break time or the next meal? Do you crave sugar and sweet things? Do you find yourself snacking to keep going? Do you suddenly run out of steam? Are you frequently tense, worried and low without good reason? These are all common symptoms of low blood sugar (hypoglycaemia) and few people realise just how quickly and easily they can be relieved.

Sugar and caffeine are not the answer

They do pick us up of course, but not for long. The tiredness comes so long after the initial lift that we never connect the coffee with the sinking feelings that follow later. But all these symptoms are largely due to the rebound effect of refined sugar and stimulants. By removing them from your diet you can rapidly recover much of your strength and stamina.

The symptoms of sugar blues listed on the next page are all so common nowadays that we struggle on regardless, little knowing how easy it can be to put things right. Somehow we never get round to doing all we intend to do, we accomplish little in a day. We may have little inclination to do anything constructive after work or school and spend hours watching television. We find ourselves in the grip of a slow and insidious inertia.

Sugar blues can be treated

These symptoms are frequently just the result of persistently low blood sugar levels, and you can revive yourself very

SUGAR BLUES

Are you . . .
Mysteriously tired?
Tense and easily stressed?
Irritable, grumpy and low?
Do you often fall asleep in the evenings?
Are you sometimes drowsy or light-headed
at the wheel of your car?

* * *

Do you crave sugar at times?
Do you lack energy and enthusiasm?
Is it hard to concentrate?
Do you daydream?
Are you a worrier?
Is life flat, dull and empty?
Is it unaccountably bleak and lonely at times?

* * *

Are you an under-achiever?
Are you mysteriously unproductive?
Is it hard to get up?
Are you often late?
Is it hard to meet deadlines?

**THIS IS THE BEGINNING OF
HYPOGLYCAEMIA**
It can be relieved

considerably with the Hay diet and blood sugar control. Many people recover their interest and enthusiasm very quickly indeed, often in a matter of days, but the symptoms are likely to return if you slip back into bad habits. Many of us can only be as efficient as we would like to be on a completely natural diet.

THAT SINKING FEELING

In 1924, in the early days of treating diabetes with insulin, a young American GP named Dr Seale Harris made a brilliant observation: that non-diabetics also suffered 'hypo' attacks of low blood sugar. He devised a diet to control the symptoms of hypoglycaemia and published his findings. But although it has long been recognised by nutritional therapists, naturopaths, and others working in complementary medicine, hypoglycaemia is still not medically accepted. Doctors are still not being trained to recognise it and, like everyone else, most still believe that sugar is the answer. Fortunately, however, this is largely a problem we can deal with ourselves.

If you suffer from Sugar Blues

Take this as a warning, your system is having trouble coping with sugar and stimulants. Gradually cut them out and replace them with natural drinks and frequent snacks of natural food. There is no other way to recover.

IS THIS YOU, TOO?

- Do you wake in the early hours of the morning, unable to get back to sleep?
- Do you wake tired or with a headache and find it improves after breakfast?
- Does an hour's shopping drain you?
- Do you need a drink after work to help you relax?

THIS IS A 'HYPO' ATTACK

A sudden drop in blood sugar levels
A dizzy, sinking feeling
Sudden intense hunger
Intense cravings for sugar
Sudden tiredness
Anxiety, tension
Blurred vision
Difficulty focusing your mind

More severe attacks
Sweating, shaking
A racing heart
Fear, panic attacks
Mood swings
A sudden feeling of nausea or illness

These attacks can leave you tired and washed out for hours
You can learn to prevent them

**AN ATTACK LIKE THIS CAN HAPPEN AT
ANY TIME**
People everywhere are having hypo attacks
Whilst driving
When operating machinery
They can even wake you in the night
They are a delayed reaction to sugar and stimulants

Blood sugar problems can run in families

Many people inherit a tendency towards hypoglycaemia and it
can show itself in many different health problems:

Diabetes	Migraine
Chronic mental illness	Eating disorders
Chronic asthma	Addictions
Hay fever	Obesity
Chronic fatigue	M.E.

Healthy people can take or leave sugar, but if your family history is like this, you could well find yourself becoming hooked on junk food. You may have to keep strictly to natural food if you are to stay well.

MAKING THE CONNECTION
I've been depressed ever since I had my baby, I get palpitations and panic attacks, I feel sick and dizzy. All my life I've had to eat little and often, otherwise my head swims and I can't concentrate. I find driving very difficult at times. Low blood sugar? That fits, there are several diabetics in our family.

ARE YOU ALLERGIC?

Allergic reactions also trigger blood sugar swings:

- Histamine in the blood triggers allergic reactions.
- When blood sugar levels are low, histamine is high, so allergic reactions are much more likely to happen.

These reactions have an effect similar to caffeine: they cause blood sugar swings, they stress the adrenal glands, filling us with tiredness and tension. Minor allergies can sometimes clear up once low blood sugar is treated.

Chronic allergies and low blood sugar go together

Allergic people, especially children, are particularly at risk from today's junk food diet. Their adrenal glands are already so overworked from dealing with constant allergic reactions that they can soon become exhausted. Every illness hits them hard; they are always tired, nervous, stressed and run down, and they are likely to need much more sleep and rest than other people. An all-natural diet can lighten the load tremendously.

Is there a test for low blood sugar?

Single blood sugar tests are of little significance. It takes a six-hour glucose tolerance test to diagnose hypoglycaemia. But the result requires expert interpretation by someone experienced in treating it, usually a naturopath or a doctor who is nutritionally orientated, and the significance of even this is disputed.

USUALLY NO TEST IS NEEDED

Low blood sugar is so easy to recognise by looking at your diet and your symptoms, and the effect of cutting out sugar and stimulants is so rapid and so convincing, that expensive testing is unnecessary for the vast majority of people. If your diet is poor, the effect of the Hay diet and blood sugar control can be dramatic.

CHRONIC HYPOGLYCAEMIA

If low blood sugar is not recognised and dealt with in the early stages it can lead to more serious mental and physical illness. Yet you will be very surprised indeed at how many of your symptoms can improve or disappear altogether, sometimes in just a few days, and the improvement will continue.

The longer you suffer, the more symptoms you accumulate

Naturally, if you have been ill for a long time it takes longer to recover, but you can still obtain considerable relief in quite a short space of time.

THIS IS CHRONIC HYPOGLYCAEMIA

Constant hunger	Constant tiredness
Midnight snacking	Tension
Headaches	PMT, menopausal problems
Irritability	Poor concentration
Mood swings	Forgetfulness
Palpitations, panics	Dizziness
Sleeping problems	Mental tiredness
Nightmares	Hormone problems
Hot or cold sweats	Depression
Night sweats	Nervousness
Itching, crawling sensations	Numbness, tingling
Cold hands and feet	Apprehension
Neck and shoulder tension	Emotional problems
Cramps of all kinds	Drowsiness
Muscle weakness	Fainting, blackouts
Chronic indigestion	Constant worrying
Menstrual cramps	Crying spells
Allergies	Chronic wheezing, asthma
Eating problems	Ringing in the ears
Chest pains	Low sex drive
Breathlessness	Sugar cravings
Muscle tension generally	Neck and shoulder tension

Routine medical tests usually prove negative

How can it cause so many different symptoms?

The brain and nervous system run on glucose. The rest of the body can burn fat or even protein for fuel if necessary, but glucose is the only fuel the brain can use, and it requires a steady, second-by-second supply of it—nothing else will do. The symptoms occur when blood sugar is low and body and mind are starved of glucose.

Are you anaemic?

The oxygen-carrying capacity of the red blood cells depends on having sufficient iron. Glucose and oxygen burn together in body cells to produce energy.

LOW BLOOD SUGAR AND ME

Like millions of other people I suffered tiredness and tension all my life. I was always stressed, I had little confidence, and over the years it grew worse, but like everyone else I struggled on. I had always wanted to write but I just never had the concentration and I assumed my many problems had nothing to do with low blood sugar since I never take sugar or caffeine. Years went by before I finally realised that my overall carbohydrate intake was so low that I too was suffering from devastating hypoglycaemia. Getting it under control has changed my life completely; my concentration improved dramatically and the relief from tension and depression was enormous. Physically I am stronger now, and more positive than I would ever have thought possible.

SEVERE HYPOGLYCAEMIA

Hypoglycaemia is a major cause of mental illness. Even at this stage, however, it can be treated, and the results can be surprisingly good. You can still improve the quality of your life, though it requires much patience and self-discipline. You also need expert help and investigation because there may be other reasons for these symptoms.

Keep very strictly to natural food

Low blood sugar is due to the unbalancing effect of sugar and processed foods on body chemistry, and very often it will have become so severely unbalanced by this time that only an

---

**THESE ARE SYMPTOMS OF SEVERE
HYPOGLYCAEMIA**

Severe panic attacks	Agoraphobia
Loss of appetite, nausea	Nightmares
Stubborn weight problems	Aggression
Neurological problems	Severe depression
Eating disorders	Anxiety neurosis
Addictions	Phobias
Migraine	Alcoholism
Severe exhaustion	Convulsions

---

entirely natural diet will be tolerated. Processed foods are so unbalanced in themselves that even a small amount may cause trouble. Food intolerances and possibly a chronic candida infection may also be involved by this stage, and the balance of the diet needs to be checked. Nevertheless, patient dieting plus vitamin and mineral supplements produce a continuing improvement.

The complicated nature of severe low blood sugar problems means that you really need professional investigation. A nutritional therapist or naturopath can help, and the services of a nutritionally orientated doctor are now becoming much easier to obtain in the UK through the health services. See 'Useful Addresses' at the end of this book.

Mercury sensitivity

People in desperate situations like this very often have large numbers of dental fillings consisting of amalgam, gold and various other metals including nickel. In addition to the problems caused by mercury, mixed metals in the mouth react with each other and greatly increase the risk of health problems of every kind (see chapter 16).

What causes
blood sugar swings ?

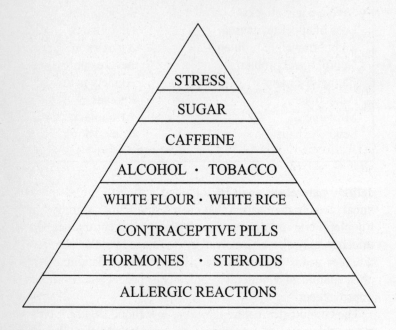

Drugs can also contribute to hypoglycaemia

They include:

- The contraceptive pill.
- Hormone replacement therapy (HRT).
- Psychiatric drugs and steroids.

ARE YOU TAKING LONG-TERM ANTIDEPRESSANTS, TRANQUILLISERS OR STEROIDS?

Drug dependence can often be reduced—but be very careful!

Powerful drugs like this, taken long term, can seriously weaken our natural healing mechanism, making the road to recovery longer and much more challenging, so wait until you have considerably recovered your strength before attempting to cut them down.

Any drastic reduction in drugs could put you in a desperate state

If you have severe nutritional problems and the drugs are reduced too quickly, the underlying illness is exposed and all the symptoms suddenly come flooding back, along with new and frightening symptoms which have developed under cover of the drugs. It could set you back a long way and leave you with worse problems than ever. So keep in close touch with your GP and consult a doctor who specialises in nutritional medicine, too, if you can. Keep yourself feeling as well as possible. I reduced my own antidepressant very gently, with the aid of a nail file.

WARNING: The sudden withdrawal of steroid drugs can be life-threatening.

A SYMPTOM GUIDE TO LOW BLOOD SUGAR

All these can be helped by the Hay diet and blood sugar control

Acidity and indigestion. Heartburn, indigestion, and the symptoms of hiatus hernia and stomach ulcers all respond exceptionally well.

Undue stress. Stress lowers blood sugar, too, which explains why some of us are constantly hungry when we are under pressure and why people who suffer from low blood sugar are so easily stressed.

Irritability, mood swings, aggression. When body chemistry is severely unbalanced it can have a deeply disturbing effect on our behaviour and emotions. When blood sugar levels are very low indeed, the brain is starved of oxygen and more basic survival behaviour can take over.

Unexplained blackouts and fainting. Dramatic symptoms like this can happen when blood sugar is critically low. Fits have also been known to occur after a sudden drop in blood sugar.

Eating disorders. Professionals who treat eating disorders are finding that they are frequently rooted in addiction to sugar and junk food.

Chronic asthma and wheezing. The tremendous increase in chronic asthma is strongly linked to the enormous rise in sugar consumption, especially amongst children, because low blood sugar increases the tendency to allergy. People often wake wheezing in the night when blood sugar levels are at their lowest. Much more can be done for asthma than most people realise by using the Hay diet and blood sugar control in addition to the usual medical treatment.

Nervous symptoms. Because glucose is the only fuel the brain can use, it is extremely sensitive to sudden changes in blood sugar levels. Nervous symptoms can sometimes be surprisingly easy to control once you understand hypoglycaemia.

Chronic mental illness. Hypoglycaemia can play a large part in anything from neurosis to psychosis and schizophrenia. Many people who suffer this way depend heavily on sugar and caffeine, convenience foods, tobacco and alcohol.

Depression. Low blood sugar is a common cause of unexplained depression.

Maturity onset diabetes. Today's hypoglycaemic often proves to be tomorrow's diabetic.

Difficulty focusing, blurred vision. The retina of the eye depends entirely on a steady and even supply of glucose for fuel. Like the brain, this is the only fuel it can use.

Headaches and migraine. The overnight drop in blood sugar levels causes some people to wake up with a headache.

Hormone problems—PMT menopausal symptoms. Many of the symptoms of PMT and the menopause are also symptoms of low blood sugar, and may therefore respond to the Hay diet and blood sugar control.

LOW BLOOD SUGAR IS A HORMONE PROBLEM
Sugar, caffeine and alcohol can upset our hormone balance

Glands are organs of the body which secrete hormones straight into the bloodstream. The pancreas is therefore a gland and insulin is a pancreatic hormone. When one gland is not working as it should, it throws the others out of balance, too. But they can very soon slip back into harmony with each other once blood sugar levels are back under control.

Muscle weakness. Muscle fatigue is greater when blood sugar is low. Some glucose is stored in the muscles, so when blood sugar is constantly at rock bottom it can leave you physically very weak indeed. But your strength soon returns if you replenish yourself with plenty of complex carbohydrate, especially fruit and whole grains.

Neurological symptoms—nerve pains. Hypoglycaemia can produce nerve pains and neurological problems of all kinds, including pins and needles, numbness, twitching and jerking of the muscles. Usually no cause can be found on medical examination.

Poor circulation. The brain takes priority when the supply of glucose is low. The blood supply to other parts of the body may therefore have to be reduced, sometimes causing muscle cramps, angina-like pain, or cold hands and feet.

HYPOGLYCAEMIA IS INVOLVED IN MANY OTHER
COMMON COMPLAINTS
It is really only an expression of unbalanced body chemistry. Oxygen is carried to the tissues by the red blood cells and it burns with glucose in body cells to release energy. So where there is a lack of glucose there is also a lack of oxygen.

CHAPTER 5

Low Blood Sugar Explained

The effect of refined sugar and stimulants depends on the adaptability and resilience of the liver and pancreas. They cause problems in susceptible people because they put the body in situations it was never designed to handle, creating tremendous internal stress. Refined sugar of all kinds is so far removed from the natural sugar beet or sugar cane that it no longer bears any resemblance to any natural food at all and, like tobacco, it can have slow, insidious and unpredictable effects. The human body had never encountered so much of it before the sugar refineries came into existence, and our general health has been deteriorating steadily ever since. If what is now known about sugar applied to any other additive, it would be banned. In days gone by, when sugar was expensive, people used it only as a spice.

What happens when we eat sugar?

Sugar shock! Instant chaos. If we suffer from hypoglycaemia, the blood sugar soars to dangerously high levels. Then a rush of insulin sends it crashing down again. It drops so low that we have to get emergency help from the adrenal glands. They pump out the stress hormones, including adrenaline, releasing sugar into the bloodstream from stores in the liver. The heart beats faster and the blood pressure goes up in a desperate bid to supply the brain with enough fuel to prevent an insulin coma— and stress and panic are the side-effects for many of us.

The effect of sugar is like revving up a car, then suddenly slamming on all the brakes. If we do it too often we are in trouble. Caffeine, alcohol and tobacco all cause similar chaos and disruption. They can eventually exhaust the pancreas, leading to diabetes, or exhaust the adrenal glands, making us increasingly tired and stressed, frequently leading to chronic fatigue and severe hypoglycaemia.

THERE ARE NO 'GOOD SUGARS'

Avoid:
White sugar, brown sugar
Raw cane sugar
Glucose and fructose
Honey

* * *

Sugar must be extracted from whole foods within our own body, not in the sugar refinery

---

But surely glucose is blood sugar!

True, but it is the form in which we take the sugar that decides whether it is good or bad; it is the source of the glucose that counts. We are not designed to handle sugar once it has been taken out of the plant.

So what is the best source of glucose?
The body must be allowed to extract its own sugar and glucose from whole foods in their natural state—from whole fruits, whole grains, salad and vegetables, including dried pulses.

Rebound hunger
Insulin and natural whole foods work together in perfect harmony. The slow and even rate at which the body extracts its own sugar from natural foods like whole grains stimulates exactly the right amount of insulin to keep blood sugar levels steady. But refined sugars are absorbed so unnaturally fast that

there is insulin left over in the bloodstream, where it carries on working, pushing blood sugar levels down below normal, and triggering rebound hunger in a vicious cycle.

Inner harmony
Natural sugar is absorbed from natural whole foods very gradually indeed, giving us a slow, time-released supply of energy which keeps us on an even keel mentally and physically. The brain and nervous system specifically require this even and controlled supply of blood sugar in order to maintain mental stability and good concentration.

HOW MUCH SUGAR IS TOO MUCH?

Before refined sugar came in, nature limited our sugar intake automatically. We would have to chew our way through at least four apples in order to get the eight teaspoonfuls of sugar often found in one can of cola. That's how unnaturally concentrated it is and how easily we can overdose on it.

Nature packages sugar

Unlike sugar, a whole food like an apple gives us very much more than just empty calories. Besides natural sugar it contains water, fibre to slow its absorption, plus just the right amount of vitamins and minerals necessary to ensure its perfect digestion. In addition, the other natural ingredients in an apple help us to function better in many different ways. By contrast, refined sugar gives us nothing but trouble. The vitamins and minerals which come with it naturally have been stripped away in the refinery. That means they have to be taken from body stores, draining our energy and creating multiple vitamin and mineral deficiencies. Sugar is also a common cause of digestive problems.

REFINED SUGAR IS REALLY JUST A CHEMICAL ADDITIVE

Sugar cane and sugar beet are the original whole plants, and they are of course natural, but only the sweet juice is squeezed out to make sugar, the rest of the plant is discarded. The juice is then heated until it crystallises, by which time all the vitamins and minerals have been processed out of it, and it contains no nutrients whatsoever. What remains is really no more than a chemical additive—and our average consumption of it is around one kilo (two pounds) per week! A hypo attack is easy to understand when you consider that a bar of chocolate, a can of cola, or even a cup of very sweet tea, delivers a blast of sugar many times more concentrated than any known natural whole food. We are consuming dangerous amounts of sugar.

ARTIFICIAL SWEETENERS
are found in:
Sports drinks

Diet foods and drinks
Low calorie, lite, sugar-free

These are artificial sweeteners too:
Aspartame
Thaumatin in confectionery
Acesulphame K in desserts and drinks

WHAT ABOUT ARTIFICIAL SWEETENERS?

They, too, are chemical additives and allergic reactions to them are not uncommon. You never really lose the taste for sugar unless you also give up artificial sweeteners. And they can sometimes trigger blood sugar swings in susceptible people.

Once you have given up sugar and artificially sweetened foods altogether, your taste buds soon wake up to all the fresh and exciting flavours of natural food. You can taste the natural sweetness in a parsnip, an onion, and even in rice. But you do have to keep strictly to natural food to appreciate it. It can sometimes take just one square of chocolate to take the taste for natural food right away again. Many people find that junk food actually tastes like junk after some time without it! I did myself.

EXACTLY HOW DOES CAFFEINE LOWER BLOOD SUGAR?

First of all it overstimulates the adrenal glands—we get a sudden surge of adrenaline. The blood pressure goes up, the heart beats faster, more sugar is released into the bloodstream and we are revived, but not for long. The sugar triggers the release of more insulin, the blood sugar level drops again and if we have hypoglycaemia we are back in a vicious cycle yet again, tired out and impatient for another fix. The overall effect of stimulants is to lower energy and raise anxiety.

What about tobacco?

Nicotine overstimulates the adrenal glands in a similar way, causing blood sugar swings. Blood sugar drops, triggering the craving for another cigarette. It's a never-ending story.

And what about alcohol?

Alcohol is actually the most refined carbohydrate of all. It lowers blood sugar by restricting the release of glucose from the liver, and it is low blood sugar that actually causes the hangover. An understanding of hypoglycaemia makes sense of the confusion, aggression, blackouts, and all the other effects of drinking too much alcohol.

87

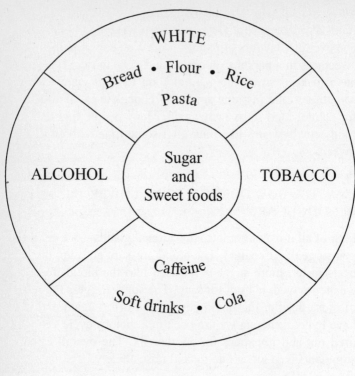

WHITE
Bread • Flour • Rice
Pasta

Sugar
and
Sweet foods

ALCOHOL

TOBACCO

Caffeine
Soft drinks • Cola

LIVING DANGEROUSLY

REFINED STARCHES LOWER BLOOD SUGAR, TOO

White bread, white rice and white flour are also quick-release carbohydrates. They, too, are unnaturally concentrated by the refining process, and turn to concentrated sugar in the body, causing more blood sugar swings.

These are all refined starches

White bread and white flours: White wheatflour, cornflour, potato flour, tapioca flour, sago flour. White flour is stripped of essential oils, vitamins, minerals and many other nutrients, so that little more than the protein (gluten) and starch remain.
White pasta: Spaghetti, noodles, pasta shapes.
Instant porridge, tapioca, sago, white semolina.
Children's breakfast cereals are usually highly processed and loaded with sugar.
Puffed grains of any kind are too refined: puffed wheat for example.
White rice: Rice flakes, ground rice, puffed rice, rice cakes.
Pearl barley.

SO WHAT'S WRONG WITH WHITE RICE?
All the vitamins and minerals are in the husk which is removed in the polishing process, so like all other highly refined foods it is dead, deficient, it cannot sustain us. If you plant a grain of white rice it will not grow, but brown rice will. White rice also contributes to a deficiency of the B vitamins in particular, resulting in tiredness and mental symptoms. Finally, it can cause blood sugar swings in much the same way that white flour does.

Whole grains are the most sustaining source of blood sugar

The sugar that the body extracts from whole grains consists of long and complex chains of molecules, which take very much longer to digest. These are the complex carbohydrates. Nature's slow and elaborate digestion is so essential because sugar must be extracted *slowly* and released *gradually* and *evenly* into the bloodstream if we are to keep stable mentally and physically.

HITTING THE WALL

The liver converts glucose to glycogen, which is body starch, and keeps it in reserve. A healthy liver can store enough for about 24–48 hours and can convert it back to glucose as needed. So we need to eat regularly to maintain our reserves, ready for whenever we need a quick burst of energy. When a marathon runner 'hits the wall' and collapses from exhaustion, his starch reserve has been drained and his blood sugar level is at rock bottom. Many athletes 'carbo-load'—they fill up on pasta and rice for a day or two before a race to make sure that they don't run out of energy.

Sudden exhaustion

Victims of severe hypoglycaemia frequently become exhausted after very little effort, because they are not very good at storing starch—they are like a battery that cannot hold a charge. To make sure you do not run out of steam it can help to have a starchy snack before and after any kind of exercise. Stamina does improve as you recover.

STUDY THE NATURAL WAY

The caffeine and junk-food habit actually impairs brain function. You will find that fresh mixed fruit blended together with water as a drink, or an apple, or a starchy snack, can pick you up almost instantly when you are mentally tired. They keep your head much clearer, too, and your mind more sharply focused. The Hay diet and blood sugar control can bring a surprising improvement in concentration and mental functioning.

ARE YOU TAKING TOO MUCH SALT?

It can damage your kidneys!

Like sugar, salt is naturally present in many foods, especially in fish, meat and vegetables, but only in very small amounts. And like refined sugar, table salt is unnaturally concentrated. It is not part of a whole food; it is therefore a chemical additive, and taking too much of it overworks the kidneys which have to excrete it, and may eventually damage them.

HOW MUCH SALT ARE YOU ACTUALLY HAVING?

Look on food packages for the salt content. The main ingredient is put first, and the others are listed in descending order of quantity. And if you consult *E for Additives* by Maurice Hanssen, and look up sodium, you will find a very long list of all the sodium compounds, such as monosodium glutamate, which are also being added to processed foods of all kinds, so you may be having more sodium than you think.

Our primitive ancestors ate mainly fresh fruit and vegetables, all rich in potassium. Salt was hard to come by, so we are naturally designed to retain the sodium and excrete the potassium in the urine with ease. But nowadays we get more salt than some of us can handle, and not nearly enough potassium from fresh fruit, vegetables and salad. This gradually changes the chemical balance of our body from its natural alkaline state to acid, making us irritable, run-down, and more susceptible to infection. The highest incidence of disease is among those who eat the least fresh fruit and vegetables.

TOO MUCH SALT CAN ALSO CAUSE BLOOD SUGAR SWINGS

Salt is a stimulant, a stressor. It causes potassium to be lost in the urine. Blood sugar levels then drop, stimulating the adrenal glands to push the blood sugar up again, making susceptible people tired and stressed. Even more potassium is lost as a result, and blood sugar levels fall again in the usual vicious cycle.

DO YOU ADD SALT TO VEGETABLES WHEN BOILING THEM?
Salt draws precious potassium out of the vegetables and into the cooking water.

SALT CAN ALSO BE VERY ADDICTIVE.
Giving it up can be very difficult indeed, and you may find, as I did at first, that the craving comes back if you have any salt at all. The salt in natural whole foods is naturally diluted, so by cutting out processed food, the Hay diet limits salt automatically, as nature does.

ARE YOU DEFICIENT IN ZINC?
If you cannot taste your food and get no enjoyment from it, you may be interested to know that loss of the sense of taste is typical of zinc deficiency, and if this is the cause it can soon be restored, and you may no longer have to load your food with salt (see p. 204).

ARE YOU BECOMING ADDICTED?

Everyday addictions are more common than we realise. Addiction is a dependence on a destructive and habit-forming substance. These things create an unnatural need; they make life a see-saw existence, full of highs and lows. Healthy people can take or leave sugar and stimulants in moderation, their body chemistry readjusts itself automatically. But in certain susceptible people—and experts suggest it could be as many as one in ten—caffeine, refined carbohydrates, sugar and sweet things, especially soft drinks, can be powerfully addictive.

BUT YOU ARE DEFINITELY NOT THE ILLNESS!
Addictions are always the result of severely unbalanced body chemistry; they have absolutely nothing to do with lack of will-power or character defects. Cravings and addictions of all kinds can be greatly relieved by the Hay diet and blood sugar

control. They are due to long-term overload with sugar and stimulants.

What is your fix?

Is is coffee, chocolate, cola, a drink, a cigarette?

- Are you constantly in need of a stimulant of some kind?
- Do you need it more and more often?
- Are you washed out and craving for another 'fix' within a very short time?
- Do you need stronger tea or coffee as time goes by?
- Do you crave sugar intensely at times?
- Do you wake in the night to snack?
- Do you drink large amounts of cola?
- Can just one biscuit lead to a binge?
- Do you need more and more chocolate to keep you going?
- Do you feel low again not long after you have put your cigarette out?
- Do you need coffee or a cigarette the moment you wake in the morning?
- Do you get frantic if you run out of your fix? Is there no way you can get through the day without it? Is the craving uncontrollable at times? Does it dominate your thoughts?

We get hooked on sugar and stimulants just to relieve the withdrawal symptoms—the slump in energy and concentration and the stress that they create. Then we take more, and the cycle is repeated. An addict's diet may eventually come to consist almost entirely of addictive substances.

Early recognition of an addictive tendency is vital

This is because severe addictions are so difficult to deal with; an addict is very often the last person to realise he has a problem at all. His habit comes before everything else, it gives him no peace, it controls his life.

ADDICTION BEGINS EARLY

Our children's diets have never been so bad. They are often tired and find it difficult to concentrate. Teaching has never been so stressful. Many teenagers are well and truly hooked on cola and chocolate, and they have easy access to them at school. *Even small children are becoming addicted*, especially to soft drinks and fruit squashes, and we do not recognise it. The more they have the more they want. Many are continually thirsty and pass lots of urine, but on all-natural drinks they soon return to drinking normally.

ADDICTION TO NATURAL FOODS

You can even become addicted to natural foods if you are aller-gic to them. Milk and wheat are the most common culprits. They, too, can unbalance body chemistry, causing blood sugar swings in the same way that junk food and caffeine do. For more about this see chapter 9.

―――― *SUGAR AND ALCOHOL—PARTNERS IN CRIME* ――――

They are BOTH refined carbohydrates.
They are both destructive

Many of us are bingeing heavily on sweet foods and soft drinks, especially cola, little knowing the dangers. People who would never abuse alcohol because they know the risks are overdosing on sugar, never seriously suspecting it could do them any real harm because its effects come on so much more slowly. Teenage delinquency is very often rooted in addiction: to sugar, alcohol and tobacco in particular. A young person may consume several litres of cola a day, and blackouts are not uncommon as a result. *Food, Teens and Behaviour* by Barbara Reed, a probation officer, gives a vivid account of her work with young people whom she was able to help by investigating their body chemistry, correcting it with vitamins and minerals where necessary, and putting them on a natural diet. Those who proved to have nutritional problems did not re-offend provided they kept to their diets.

Natural Justice is an organisation committed to this approach. The address is at the end of the book.

THIS IS THE TRAGEDY
Addiction to junk foods and stimulants can set the scene for drug addiction. Many young people with sugar blues feel hopeless and inadequate, they do not understand why they cannot keep up with the others. They suffer in silence, sometimes to the point where it becomes difficult to cope with everyday life. Teenage suicides are not uncommon. Yet young people especially can recover astonishingly quickly once sugar and stimulants are cut out and they are established on regular meals of natural food.

GIVING UP ONE ADDICTION CAN LEAD TO ANOTHER
Many people who give up smoking come to depend on sweets or coffee for the lift they got from tobacco. Alcohol, tobacco, sugar and caffeine all have to go eventually. You will not completely solve your problem until you have given them all up. Improving your diet makes the cravings very much easier to deal with.

How Celia finally conquered tobacco

Celia found the Hay diet and blood sugar control difficult at first, but after five weeks' hard work she was jubilant. 'Have I got news for you! I've given up smoking—after ten years. I've tried everything. Now I know I'll never go back to it.' And four months later she was still not smoking. 'When I gave up coffee I found I didn't need the cigarettes. I'd never tried giving up coffee and cigarettes together before, and I'm sure I couldn't have given up one without the other. Nowadays I find coffee tastes like poison.'

95

There were other benefits too

Celia had always felt she was too thin, she could never put on weight, but now she's put on a stone (14 pounds) and she is delighted. Her hair has thickened up 'like a mop', and her skin, always soggy in the bath, is waterproof since taking evening primrose oil. And there's more: she's more energetic, much less stressed, and thinking of taking up new hobbies.

You name it, Ralph had it!

Ralph was taking a litre of indigestion mixture every week. He had persistent sore throats and difficulty in swallowing. He had chest pains and he was short of breath. After many tests and examinations, all negative, a locum GP asked about his diet and lifestyle. He was a smoker and he was eating and drinking from the vending machine at work—cola, coffee, chocolate bars, one thing led to another! 'You are being poisoned by sugar,' said the doctor.

'It had to go,' said Ralph, and he gave it up without hesitation. He gave up sugar, white bread, coffee and tobacco all at the same time. Within a week he felt very much better and he soon got back to normal. Nowadays he looks exceptionally fit, plays lots of sport, and is very enthusiastic about his new lifestyle.

CHAPTER 6

Blood Sugar Control

There is still a lot of confusion over how low blood sugar should be treated. When I was teaching the Hay diet, nine out of ten people on every course were suffering from hypoglycaemia to some extent, and most mistakenly believed sugar to be the answer. But remember, we can get all the sugar we need from fresh fruits and vegetables, and because the body also extracts sugar from whole grains, we don't need refined sugar at all.

Keep to the Hay diet

It ensures the best possible results in the shortest possible time. It stabilises blood sugar levels because it consists of the whole and balanced foods so necessary to restore and maintain our natural equilibrium.

- Gradually reduce sugar and stimulants.
- Eat regularly—never miss a meal.
- Snack between meals if necessary.
- You may need more than one starch meal a day.
- Remember that caffeine, alcohol and tobacco also disrupt blood sugar levels.

When do I get results?

Usually in a very few days. Many people recover quickly and can control their blood sugar without further measures. Such rapid improvements in the quality of life may come as a great surprise. But if you have suffered a long time you will need to work at it. After an initial lift, the improvement continues more slowly, over weeks and months.

Change your diet slowly

Blood sugar control has to be learnt, it takes time and patience. Naturally, when you first discover you have low blood sugar you will want to cut out all the sugar and stimulants without delay, but be careful. Cut them down slowly, especially if you have been taking them in large amounts, and replace them with natural foods and drinks which you enjoy. Sudden drastic changes in diet can sometimes leave a debilitated person feeling very weak indeed, so give yourself time to adapt, keep yourself feeling as well as possible. If you do suffer initially make sure you replenish yourself with plenty of natural food, especially whole grains with pulses. Concentrated protein like meat also helps stabilise blood sugar levels, and your strength will gradually return over the next few days.

Withdrawal symptoms include tiredness, lightheadedness, headaches and stomach pains, but not everybody gets withdrawal symptoms.

DO YOU CRAVE SUGAR?

The Hay diet and blood sugar control can put an end to the most intense cravings in many people. But if you still crave sugar despite these measures, read on. Severe cravings for sugar, alcohol, bread and yeast may point to candida (see chapter 7).

- Dilute concentrated fruit juices, otherwise they may cause blood sugar swings.
- Decaffeinated tea and coffee are a compromise because they are chemically processed.

CAFFEINE IS A POWERFUL ADDICTIVE DRUG

As explained in chapter 5, it lifts you up but it can let you down badly, leaving you washed out and desperate for yet another fix. Few people realise what caffeine is doing to them.

WHAT CAN I DRINK?

Water
Herbal teas
Pure fruit juices
not 'Fruit Juice Drinks'
Sparkling water with a slice of lemon
Decaffeinated tea or coffee

ALL SUBSTANCES WHICH DISRUPT BLOOD
SUGAR LEVELS MUST EVENTUALLY BE KEPT
OUT OF THE DIET

There is no other way to recover

Reduce caffeine slowly

If you are drinking a lot of tea or coffee, cut it down slowly enough to minimise withdrawal symptoms. You may get a headache or a light head, so be careful when driving. You may also get a reaction when you try it again—any symptoms at all, including stomach pains, a headache perhaps, or you may suddenly feel faint.

- Percolated coffee is highest in caffeine.
- Decaffeinated coffee helps many people, but it does contain other stimulants besides caffeine, and it can still cause stomach acidity.
- Avoid stewed tea: removing the teabag from the teapot once it is ready to drink limits the caffeine content.
- Decaffeinated teabags taste like ordinary tea.

ARE YOU DRINKING TOO MUCH TEA OR COFFEE?

Are you . . .
Tired, tense,
stressed, sleepless?
Anxious, nervous, shaky,
grumpy, irritable?
Does it make your heart race?

Important decisions are being taken on little else but coffee!

* * *

THE LIMIT PER DAY
2 cups of coffee
or 4 cups of tea
Caffeine and sugar together are double trouble

* * *

These contain caffeine too:
Cola drinks, cocoa, chocolate
Some of the painkillers
Healthy people can take limited amounts of caffeine

Caffeine makes you thirsty

- It is partly its addictive nature which makes us crave more.
- It is dehydrating because it is a diuretic; it makes us pass more urine.

Once you have cut it out you will notice that you need to drink less often. Sleeping problems can sometimes improve without caffeine.

100

PICK YOURSELF UP NATURALLY

Snack between meals on any natural food
Avocado pears
Firm, fresh fruits
Nuts, seeds
Natural yoghurt
Wholemeal bread or crispbreads
Raw carrot, celery sticks, salad

* * *

**Only natural foods and drinks can pick you up
without letting you down**
Time the snacks to avoid the tiredness and
flagging concentration

Fruits are ideal for a quick burst of energy because the sugar they contain is rapidly absorbed.

ARE YOU ON A RESTRICTED DIET?

Without a good understanding of low blood sugar, restricted diets for food intolerance or candida can leave you weak and sinking, perpetually depressed or in a constant state of panic. Remember that even if you never have sugar or stimulants you can still suffer from hypoglycaemia if your total intake of concentrated starch is too low. You need plenty of potatoes and grains, to maintain energy levels and keep your brain functioning properly.

A TEST FOR LOW BLOOD SUGAR

BE CAREFUL WHEN TESTING

Once you have completely cut out sugar, caffeine and the other stimulants, be very careful when you try them again for the first time, especially if you are unwell. You may get a sharp reaction.

- Headaches, stomach aches, a racing heart and faintness are not uncommon.
- Very occasionally someone may have a devastating reaction to sugar or alcohol.
- Others may react sharply to caffeine or a cigarette.

There is no need to test them at all if you are happy without them.

How long shall I have to avoid sugar and stimulants?
Keep right away from them until you feel better. Some people find that they can take them occasionally, but others can only keep well if they avoid them altogether.

HELP!

I feel more and more tired and washed out while I am preparing the evening meal.
Eat regularly through the day. Have a starchy snack before you begin.

I am too busy to eat all day. I binge when I get home.
Strict two-hourly snacks of natural whole foods can prevent bingeing. Fresh fruit and nuts are a good idea.

I wake up so tired that my husband has to bring me breakfast in bed to give me the strength to get up.
Your blood sugar drops overnight, so have a starchy snack before you go to bed and again if you wake in the early hours of the morning.

TREATING CHRONIC HYPOGLYCAEMIA

——————————*EAT TWO-HOURLY*——————————

Here are some suggestions to get you started:

STARCH SNACKS	PROTEIN SNACKS
Porridge with sunflower seeds	Apple and cheese
A firm under-ripe banana	Raw carrot and nuts
A salad sandwich	Chicken leg with salad
Hearty vegetable soup	Boiled egg with salad
Brown rice and peas or beans	Natural yoghurt with fruit
Wholemeal roll with salad	Sliced meat and salad
Wholemeal crispbreads	Fish with salad
Jacket potato with salad	Fresh fruit

Spread food out evenly over the day

Absolutely regular meals and snacks are the key to good blood sugar control. Once you are in the habit of eating two-hourly and you begin to feel the benefit, you will find that your body demands to be fed every two hours. Missing a snack can bring the symptoms back and make you very tired indeed. You may even need to carry food with you to prevent it.

Time your snacks to avoid the 'lows'
It can take a long time to work out what to eat and when. If you wait until you are sinking with hunger before you eat, it may be too late to avoid the tiredness that comes afterwards, especially if you are very unwell. But as you recover the food begins to take effect more quickly. Wholegrain foods like porridge and wholemeal bread stabilise blood sugar the most effectively. And again, fruit is best for a quick lift.

Snack according to the principles of the Hay diet

- Absolutely no processed food.
- At least 50 per cent fresh fruit, vegetables and salad.
- Cut right down on salt.
- Drink plenty of water.

Blood sugar levels always drop overnight
A substantial starchy snack before you go to bed helps you to relax. If you wake in the night and cannot get back to sleep, another starchy snack could solve the problem and you will wake feeling stronger, warmer and much less tired. You could keep a snack ready beside the bed. You should find that in time you are able to sleep for longer.

If midnight snacks are a persistent problem
You may find, as I did, that 3g of evening primrose oil per day allows you to sleep through the night without snacking. It is a good idea to increase your overall intake of the other natural oils at the same time, especially extra virgin olive oil.

Extra vitamins and minerals are required
People with chronic hypoglycaemia usually suffer from quite severe vitamin and mineral deficiencies, having run themselves down over a very long time. A stressful life also lowers blood sugar and further drains us of nutrients. You can make up the deficiencies and support your adrenal glands by following the powerful supplement programme on p. 202. You will be very surprised at the lift it gives you.

Avoid very high protein diets which are low in starch
Remember that although they can control the symptoms of hypoglycaemia, they can lead to more problems, including degenerative illness in the long term.

Make the starch meals richer and more sustaining
Eat plenty of whole grains including millet.

- Beans and peas, including dried pulses, with grains are particularly sustaining.
- A few sunflower seeds can be added to porridge.
- A little butter or extra virgin olive oil taken with whole grains also makes a meal more satisfying.

Recipes for low blood sugar
The recipes in any of the food combining recipe books are suitable for people with low blood sugar because they are all natural and sugar-free.

A vegetarian diet for low blood sugar
See *Hypoglycaemia: A Better Approach* by Dr Paavo Airola. Meat is optional. There are details of where to obtain this book in Further Reading at the end of the book.

CHAPTER 7

Candida: the Missing Diagnosis

It was during the 1970s that an American physician, Dr Orion Truss, observed that thrush infections improved very considerably when treated with a sugar-free, yeast-free diet. He also found that this diet brought dramatic relief to a huge number of other people with mysterious mental and physical symptoms of all kinds, whom he had previously been unable to help. But he failed to convince his medical colleagues that a simple fungal infection could be at the root of so many of our common complaints, so in 1982 he published *The Missing Diagnosis* to inform patients directly about candida.

Candida overgrowth is a new problem, a yeast or thrush infection of the gut caused mainly by the continuing change in our eating habits from natural food to a diet high in processed foods, especially sugar and alcohol, which feed the yeast. Fungal infections like this were rare at the beginning of the twentieth century, but today they are everywhere and can sometimes be difficult to keep in check. The main reason for medical scepticism is that candida is a natural inhabitant of the human body anyway, and only causes trouble when it gets out of control; there is therefore no completely reliable laboratory test to confirm it. The recognition and treatment of chronic candida are not part of a doctor's training, although the condition is well known to naturopaths, nutritional therapists and others working in complementary medicine.

The fact that candida is not recognised allows it to progress unhindered, and when it is neglected it can change into an aggressive fungal infection. These fungi put down threadlike roots which pierce the gut, so that candida toxins can enter the bloodstream and invade every system of the body, including the brain, causing an endless list of symptoms. Diagnosis can be difficult because it affects people in so many different ways, so possibly the best person to recognise it is yourself. The aim of this chapter is to open your eyes to candida, so that you can deal with it in the early stages, because if the diet is not

---

THIS IS CHRONIC CANDIDA

Catarrh	Headaches
Furred mouth	Depression
Thrush in the mouth	Itchy anus, vulva, vagina
Persistent sore throat	Rashes, urticaria, itching
Indigestion, stomach ache	Persistent vaginal thrush
Bloating, belching	Hot flushes
Embarrassing wind	Fatigue
Constant overheating	Difficulty keeping warm
Irritable bowel	Wheezing
Diarrhoea, constipation	Irritability
Mucus problems anywhere	Chemical sensitivity
Muscle aches	Dizziness
Chronic 'flu	Joint pain and swelling
Food intolerance	Burning anywhere
Poor immunity	Severe forgetfulness
Spots before the eyes	Watering eyes
Sore, irritable bladder	Feeling ill with tiredness
Recurrent cystitis	Pelvic infections
Endometriosis	Mental fogging
Cravings for sugar,	Premenstrual tension
bread or alcohol	(PMT)

Medical tests are usually negative

---

changed at this time it can only get worse. Diagnosis is made on your history, symptoms and response to treatment.

Candida affects men, women and children, young and old. Many people feel they have some kind of mysterious infection, and it is often a major unrecognised factor in M.E. and chronic fatigue syndrome.

LOCALISED CANDIDA INFECTIONS
Sometimes the immune system is strong enough to confine candida to one or two systems of the body, and prompt treatment can prevent further spread.

A major crisis can be the last straw

Many people can trace the onset of their illness to traumatic events in their lives. If our general health is already poor, major stresses like this can devastate our immunity, leaving us wide open to allergies, to candida and to virus infections.

Beat burn-out

Not knowing how to regenerate ourselves, we struggle on until we run our batteries right down. We become mentally and physically exhausted, and badly drained of essential nutrients: vitamins, minerals and essential natural oils. But the good news is that you can replenish yourself with the Hay diet, plus the supplement programme on p. 202. And many people recover their strength and stamina in a surprisingly short time.

CANDIDA SYMPTOM GUIDE

Oral thrush. This can sometimes be severe and very distressing. If it is persistent and the mouth alone is treated, it comes straight back from farther down the gullet, so it also needs to be treated systemically with diet and with antifungal medicines if necessary. Holding a little natural yoghurt or an antifungal preparation in the mouth can sometimes ease the pain and help to clear the infection.

───────────────*THRUSH IN THE MOUTH*───────────────

White spots	Chronic sore throat
Furred tongue	Bad taste, bad breath
Sore mouth	Burning mouth and throat
Sore, burning gullet	Difficulty swallowing

White septic pimples in the mouth and throat which never go away

The anti-candida diet speeds recovery

───

Candida and chronic asthma. Many people with severe asthma, who are very debilitated and taking long-term steroids, are victims of the most devastating candida infections. Many have suffered for years, not knowing the cause of their distress. Steroid inhalers can be associated with severe oral thrush.

Furred tongue. The tongue may be heavily furred, and can sometimes even be yellow. There may be a line down the middle, or it may be cracked all over like crazy paving. A cracked tongue indicates vitamin deficiencies, especially a lack of vitamin B complex. As your general health improves, the coating clears, the cracks heal, and the mucous membrane becomes strong, pink and healthy again.

Belching, bloating, gas and wind. Yeast in the stomach and intestines ferments with sugar or alcohol to make gas, just as it does when yeast is mixed with sugar to make bread.

Irritable bowel. This often clears up on the Hay diet alone, but candida is also commonly involved in it.

Chronic diarrhoea. Typically, candida diarrhoea bubbles and 'boils'. You can sometimes feel it fermenting in the intestine. Sugar, sweet foods and alcohol make the wind and diarrhoea worse and the bowel gas can sometimes be very offensive indeed. Very often fruit has to be cut out completely for a time, in order to recover.

Severe diarrhoea. People with severe diarrhoea and drastic loss of weight become desperate when doctors cannot stop it and the cause cannot be found. Yet powerful antifungal drugs such as Nystatin are freely available on medical prescription.

Recurrent vaginal thrush. When the gut is infected with candida, the infection travels forward again and again from anus to vagina. It obviously needs to be treated with diet in addition to the usual medical treatment, but even then it can be very stubborn. People who suffer from thrush over a long period frequently become increasingly tired and unwell because they are developing the many other symptoms of candida.

Candida can be sexually transmitted.

Candida cystitis. Repeated attacks of cystitis for which no cause can be found are often associated with vaginal thrush, but not always, for the candida infection travels forward from the vagina. Antibiotics make candida cystitis worse by killing the friendly bacteria in the gut, thereby lowering resistance to fungal infections.

Sore, irritable bladder. In addition to the anti-candida diet (see chapter 8), increasing the amount of natural oils in the diet, especially extra virgin olive oil, can provide substantial relief. They improve the condition of the mucous membrane inside the bladder, thereby reducing the soreness.

Jock itch. A maddening itch round the anus, usually in men but sometimes also in women. It can sometimes affect the vulva and vagina. Antifungal creams alone do not have any lasting effect, it has to be treated with diet as well.

Body odour. A sour, yeasty smell which does eventually clear up with candida treatment.

Skin problems:

- An itchy scalp.
- Persistent rashes of all kinds.
- A generally itchy skin or a mysterious, deep itch, when

there is no rash to be seen at all. This can sometimes be severe, preventing sleep.

Urticaria (nettle rash). These are the large whitish, itchy weals that can suddenly appear at any time, especially after eating. A severe attack can be alarming. They quickly spread over the whole body, but usually disappear without trace within twenty-four hours. People who have suffered miserably for years can sometimes find relief in candida treatment.

Psoriasis too will often respond to anti-candida treatment.

Athlete's foot and fungal infections of the nails. The nails can become very deformed indeed.

Addictions to sugar and yeast. These are frequently also related to candida. Sugar cravings can be intense. Other people find they crave bread and eat it in large quantities. Such people are frequently overweight. There also some people who have a special liking for mushrooms or yeast extract spreads like Marmite.

Mucus problems anywhere:

- A runny nose, catarrh or sinus problems.
- A post-nasal drip: mucus runs down the back of the throat at night, causing an irritating cough.
- Glue ear, ear infections, ear pain, deafness.
- Mucus in the stools.
- Mucus in the chest, causing cough, wheezing, asthma, chest infections.

Hormone problems, PMT. The symptoms of candida are often mistakenly attributed to the menopause or PMT. Sweats, hot flushes and constant overheating are also typical of candida.

Flushing or burning, absolutely anywhere. Face, mouth, stomach, gut, vagina, feet, joints—any of these may be affected. This problem is very common indeed, and it does gradually improve as you conquer candida.

Mental symptoms. Candida toxin is powerful and can affect the brain, producing mental fogging, mood swings and irritability, but it can sometimes clear up surprisingly fast with treatment. The alcohol produced when sugar and yeast ferment together in the body also contributes to mental symptoms, including depression, irritability, mood swings and severe forgetfulness.

Migraine, especially with vomiting. Lifelong sufferers can sometimes find relief in candida treatment.

Chronic flu. A serious and growing problem which is frequently due to candida. Victims are always tired, with aching limbs. They get shivering attacks, feel generally very chilly and there is a constant feeling of illness. In addition to the diet, anti-candida preparations such as caprylic acid or Nystatin can bring dramatic relief.

Food intolerances. Chronic candida can so damage the lining of the gut that it becomes porous and large molecules of partly digested food may enter the bloodstream and set up allergic reactions. Many candida victims are intolerant of wheat and dairy products. When candida is of long standing and powerful drugs have been used long term to suppress the symptoms, there are frequently multiple food sensitivities.

Other allergies. Allergies of all kinds are more troublesome if you have candida. If they are mild they can sometimes clear up with candida treatment.

Joint pains, rheumatoid arthritis. Much more can be done for arthritis of all kinds than most of us realise, if you are willing to work on your diet. It can sometimes respond dramatically to the Hay diet. Candida, too, is very commonly involved in it. The improvement has to be experienced to be believed. I would myself be crippled if I ate anything fried or browned.

Low resistance to infection. People with chronic candida may suffer frequent infections of all kinds because candida weakens our natural defences.

Diabetics are especially prone to candida because of their high blood sugar levels.

Chemical sensitivity. Candida victims frequently react to perfumes, and other chemical odours such as insecticides, plastics and tobacco smoke. Overexposure to chemical fumes can sometimes bring on a severe attack of candida.

DRUGS AND CANDIDA

Female hormones favour the growth of candida, which is why it is more common in women. High sugar diets, combined with contraceptive pills and other hormone preparations, increase the risk of candida by raising blood sugar levels. Everyday hormonal problems can stabilise very quickly on the Hay diet and blood sugar control, with treatment for candida if necessary. The contraceptive pill is a steroid hormone.

Steroids

Steroids, too, encourage candida by raising blood sugar levels. Suppressing symptoms with drugs progressively weakens your natural resistance, and many people taking long-term steroids eventually find they have severe candida and multiple allergies, especially to food. Nevertheless, you can still vastly improve the quality of your life.

WARNING: Remember that the sudden reduction or withdrawal of steroid drugs can be life-threatening. Wait until you have considerably recovered your strength, then consult your doctor about cutting them down. It is important to be aware of the side-effects of steroids.

ANTIBIOTICS ENCOURAGE CANDIDA

Antibiotics kill all bacteria, good and bad, including the friendly bacteria which keep candida under control, but they cannot destroy yeasts and fungi. So when friendly bacteria are sufficiently reduced in numbers, we are left wide open to candida. It rushes in to occupy the empty space, never missing an opportunity.

The onset of candida can be sudden, but usually it is slow and insidious

People taking long-term antibiotics, or repeated courses over a short period of time, may eventually find themselves becoming increasingly tired, with a growing list of other symptoms which they and their doctor may not connect with the antibiotic. The massive doses of antibiotics often given after an injury are another common contributor to candida.

Why are antibiotics prescribed so often?

It is partly because the role that candida and food intolerance play in recurrent infections is not being recognised, especially where there is mucus. The underlying cause of repeated chest infections, ear infections and sinus problems, for example, is frequently the mucus produced by an intolerance to dairy products, and these problems may continue indefinitely unless the allergic source of the infection is identified and removed. So the patient becomes locked into a vicious cycle of more infections and more antibiotics, growing progressively weaker and ever more susceptible to candida. Broad spectrum antibiotics are the most destructive.

Avoid antibiotics if you can

Everyday infections can sometimes be very effectively treated with the vitamin and mineral supplement programme on p. 202. If an antibiotic is essential, be sure to take natural yoghurt or acidophilus capsules at the same time, to minimise its effect on the good bacteria in the gut.

ANTIBIOTICS AND CHRONIC FATIGUE

Alan had been taking antibiotics for acne over eight months, and during this time he had become increasingly tired and aching. The problem had become so bad that he was having trouble coping with his job in computers. He rightly suspected that there might be a connection with the antibiotics, but his doctor was so completely reassuring that he carried on taking them.

He had mucus problems too, and his brain was so fogged at times that he felt he was 'not on this planet'. He was eating lots of cheese, which he decided to cut out to see it it made any difference. Without the dairy products his head and chest felt clearer and he was becoming much more resistant to infection. Six weeks later he had discontinued the antibiotic and the acne had not returned. He felt stronger, less aching and less tired. Having been without alcohol for two weeks, he felt decidedly worse after two pints of beer, so he began to suspect that he had candida. 'I've always eaten everything without worrying about it, but once you find out about complementary medicine, you wonder how anyone ever manages without it!'

CANDIDA DIARRHOEA

Ron had candida coming on over six months, with offensive bowel gas, loose stools and a gradual loss of weight. Normally an industrious man, he began sitting around and falling asleep. The last straw came when he varnished the wood panels in the bathroom, inhaling lots of fumes in an enclosed space. The diarrhoea took off with a vengeance, and he lost so much weight that he was afraid he might have cancer. He was eating far too many sweets but would not hear of changing his diet. His doctor could not solve the problem, and a bowel specialist recommended a barium enema which revealed nothing.

By now Ron was desperate enough to try anything. He cut out sugar and yeast, but although the diarrhoea did improve a lot, it did not stop. Then, after three days on an antifungal drug, it stopped altogether. He remained on the anti-candida diet and the drugs over the next three months until he had regained his normal weight, then gradually cut the drug down. Nine months later he was back to a normal diet.

MOULD SENSITIVITY

People who suffer from candida are frequently affected by moulds because yeasts and moulds are related—they are all fungi. Symptoms can appear almost immediately or they may be delayed by an hour or two. Very many people are affected by inhaled mould spores but the problem usually goes unrecognised.

ARE YOU MOULD SENSITIVE?

How do you feel in:
Jumble sales
Second-hand clothes shops
Second-hand bookshops
Auction rooms
Attics, barns, greenhouses
Damp, mouldy places

Mould spores affect some people when:
Handling compost
Walking through autumn leaves

It can cause absolutely any symptoms:
Sudden tiredness
Sweats, burning, bloating
Wheezing, depression, fainting

How do you feel on damp days?

There are more mould spores around on damp days; some people feel worse when it is raining or before a thunderstorm. If your house is particularly damp and mouldy, note how you feel when you are away.

How does it happen?

Inhaled mould spores enter the bloodstream through the lungs. As natural healing progresses, the mucous membranes heal and resistance improves.

CHAPTER 8

Treating Candida

Diet is the first line of defence: a yeast-free, sugar-free diet starves the candida bugs and they die off. But because candida only goes out of control when our immune defences are down, we cannot even begin to relax the diet until we have rebuilt our natural immunity and put our own body in a strong enough position to control candida by itself. It can take several weeks or months to get back to normal but it can sometimes be done with diet alone, even when it is quite severe. Learn all you can about the anti-candida diet and keep to it one hundred per cent because getting it wrong can keep you ill despite any other treatments.

Start with the Hay diet

It will accelerate your recovery. Make it anti-candida by cutting out the foods listed in the box opposite. Food combining reduces gut fermentation and wind, and you will definitely need 50 per cent raw vegetables and salads to heal your gut and mucous membranes.

Why cut these foods out?

- Sugar and alcohol feed the yeast.
- Yeast and fungus foods add to the problem. Bread contains yeast.
- Fermented foods like cheese also add to the problem.
- Peanuts grow in the ground and contain some powerful moulds.

THE ANTI-CANDIDA DIET

Outline only

CUT OUT:

Sugar	Melon
Yeast	Grapes and dried fruit
Alcohol	Mushrooms
White flour	Peanuts
Bread	Cheese
Yeast extract spreads	Quorn (a fungus food)
All sweetened foods	
Any other fermented foods or drinks	

RESTRICT: Milk and fruit

EVERYONE HAS TO DIET
**Other treatments alone will not cure or
control candida**
Most people keeping strictly to this diet can expect
considerable improvement in 1–4 weeks

- Milk contains milk sugar which does not taste sweet. Plain soya milk is sugar free.
- White flour turns to sugar in the body.

Change your diet slowly

Give yourself time to adapt.

1 Replace sugar and sweetened foods with fruit at first, especially if you crave sugar.
2 Replace bread with soda bread, rice and potatoes.

3   Slowly reduce alcohol.
4   Restrict fruit. Gradually replace it with raw vegetables
    and salad—avocado pears, raw carrots, red and yellow
    peppers, celery, etc.

WHAT CAN I EAT INSTEAD OF BREAD?

Have plenty of these:
Potatoes
Brown rice
Wholewheat pasta
Natural oats: porridge or muesli
Whole millet, raw buckwheat, quinoa
Soda bread is yeast-free
Wholewheat or rye crispbreads and rice cakes
(These are too light to depend on entirely)

BE CAREFUL

If you are relying mainly on whole grains and potatoes for starch, make sure you get enough to keep your blood sugar level steady. Porridge with sunflower seeds, and pulses combined with grains, are particularly sustaining.

Use wholewheat soda bread if you can

Cutting out bread altogether automatically reduces your starch intake. Soda bread is available from supermarkets, but it is usually made with white flour. Most cookbooks have a recipe for soda bread. It is easy to make and can be frozen, and it is also becoming more widely available from health food shops and some of the larger supermarkets.

Sourdough breads are not suitable because, although they do not contain yeast, they are still fermented.

Wholemeal flour can be used in cooking provided it is cooked without yeast.

You could make your own chapatis Most commercial Indian flat breads contain yeast or sugar.

WHAT CAN I DRINK?

Herbal teas
Spring water with a slice of lemon
Unsweetened soya milk
A little milk
Decaffeinated tea or coffee
(a compromise)

FRUIT AND CANDIDA

- *Cut out grapes and dried fruit.*
- *Restrict all other fruit.*
- *Avoid over-ripe fruits*: they contain yeasts and moulds, especially on the skin. Choose the firmer, less ripe fruits.
- *Over-ripe melons and very sweet yellow pears* contain a lot of sugar and yeast and can sometimes cause a flare-up of candida.
- *Grapes* can contain up to 50 per cent sugar and have yeasts and moulds on the skins. This is what ferments the grapes into wine.
- *Dried fruit.* Drying fruit concentrates the sugar up to 50 per cent. The skins also contain invisible moulds.
- *A ripe banana* can contain the equivalent of up to three tea-spoonfuls of natural sugar. The starch in a banana turns to sugar as it ripens.
- *Fruit juices.* Freshly squeezed fruit juices are best. Concentrated fruit juices need to be diluted. They also contain a lot of yeast.

You may have to cut out fruit altogether for a while

A candida bug does not know the difference between refined sugar and the natural sugar in fruit, and many candida sufferers eat fruit to excess. If your recovery is slow, you could try cutting out fruit to see if you feel better. Irritable bowel, and diarrhoea in particular, may improve without it. Many people with severe chronic candida find that even a small amount of fruit will cause it to flare up. We do not strictly need it if we are taking plenty of salad and raw vegetables.

What can I eat instead of fruit?

Make raw vegetables and salads up to at least 50 per cent of the diet.
Salad of all kinds:
Avocado pear, raw carrot, cauliflower and leek.
Cucumber, tomatoes, celery and green salad.
Avocado pear, tomatoes, celery and beetroot.
Spring onions, lettuce and radishes.
Cabbage and celeriac.
Try some of the more unusual salads:
Chicory, fennel, red, yellow and green peppers

HAY DIET MEALS FOR CANDIDA

Protein meals are no problem, except that cheese must be avoided. Ideas for starch meals are given below.

BREAKFASTS
Weetabix or shredded wheat with soya milk.
Wholewheat crispbreads with sliced tomato and cress.
Toasted soda bread with butter.
Oatmeal porridge with soya milk.
Millet flake porridge.

Avocado cream
Blend together: Half an avocado pear, water, 1 teaspoonful
extra virgin olive oil.

SNACKS
Homemade soda bread sandwiches filled with:
Hummus (chick-pea pâté).
Tahini or nut butter (not peanut).
Salad, or any other vegetarian filling.

Oatcakes, ricecakes
Open sandwiches piled with mixed salad.

MAIN MEAL SUGGESTIONS
Corn on the cob with butter.
Potato cakes made with egg yolk.
Veggieburgers.
Wholewheat pasta or rice with vegetarian sauce.
Hearty vegetable soup with soda bread.
Vegetable stews or casseroles with potato.
Savoury brown rice or any other grains mixed with fresh
vegetables and lentils or beans.
Soya milk puddings made with brown rice or millet.

Chronic candida and low blood sugar go together

People with chronic candida usually also suffer from hypoglycaemia, so they have to be treated together. After the initial lift,
you may feel worse on the anti-candida diet if you are not getting enough concentrated starch foods to keep your blood sugar
level up. You may even experience hypo attacks for the first
time, so be sure to get enough concentrated starch to fuel your
energy and keep you feeling well.

Make sure you get enough essential oils

Fat intake is usually considerably reduced on an anti-candida diet. You will need plenty of natural unrefined oils to heal and seal the gut.

A TEST FOR CANDIDA

This test is only to prove a point, it is not strictly necessary. You could use it if you are still not convinced and if you are reasonably fit. If you are very debilitated the reactions could be much more severe.

The first step

Try the anti-candida diet for at least four weeks. You need to cut out the foods as specified on the previous pages. Be very strict or it will not work.

The next step

Whenever you feel considerably better than you were before you began the diet, try the forbidden foods in small quantities, one at a time, and note the effects. Wait for any symptoms to clear before trying another food.

BE CAREFUL
Reactions can be surprisingly sharp. You could be affected for anything up to a day or two. Sugar, beer and wine can be particularly upsetting.

DELAYED REACTIONS
Once you are established on the anti-candida diet you may find that if you break it, it takes several doses of sweet food or bread to build up to a reaction, so the cause of the trouble is often hard to recognise.

RESIST TEMPTATION IF YOU POSSIBLY CAN

Few people realise how aggressive candida can be and how strict you have to be with the anti-candida diet. If you are severely affected, just one piece of cake could set you back for days. A bar of chocolate can sometimes be like pouring oil on to a fire. Be extra careful over Christmas and on holiday because relaxing the diet completely in the early stages of treatment can bring all the symptoms back and prolong the illness. Any expensive tests and treatments will then have been a waste of money, because their effects will be undone and you will be back where 'you started. Again, reactions to forbidden foods can build up over several days.

Shall I recover completely?

Most people do, eventually. Much depends on how strictly you can keep to the diet. People who have suffered for many years may need much self-discipline to keep themselves well. Every mistake in the diet and every stressful event brings a renewed assault and controlling candida becomes a way of life.

CANDIDA AND ALCOHOL

An unpleasant reaction to alcohol—to beer and wine especially—is a strong pointer to candida. Wine produces some of the fastest and worst reactions. Sweet wine, sherry and champagne are a great feast for candida bugs—sugar, yeast *and* alcohol. As mentioned above, the reaction is delayed, the connection is not easy to make; however, if you cut out alcohol altogether for a week or two you will definitely feel the difference if candida is a problem.

Reactions to beer can be so severe and so debilitating that it sometimes has to be cut out completely. And beer can also cause a lot of embarassing wind with a characteristic and very unpleasant odour. Young candida victims may find having to go without alcohol a great problem, especially at first. But most regular drinkers do give it up eventually, rather than face the consequences. They can still go out with their friends and they just drink sparkling water with a slice of lemon.

REDUCE GUT FERMENTATION AND WIND
(*belching and bowel gas*)

What causes it?

- All the foods forbidden on the anti-candida diet, especially sugar and alcohol.
- Constipation—keep the bowel clear.
- Too much meat.
- Too much fruit.
- Overeating generally.
- Incompatible mixtures of food.
- Soya milk in some cases. Because it is made from beans, some people react to it with bloating and wind.

If you are very sensitive to mould you may also be affected by:

Beanshoots	Sprouted seeds
Commercial ground spices	Dried herbs
Herbal teas	Nuts and seeds

Whole spices, fresh herbs and nuts in shells will probably be all right.

Peel all root vegetables—there is mould on the skins.

- Scrub potatoes before you scrape or peel them.
- Do not eat the skin of jacket potatoes.

Avoid very old potatoes. Sometimes at the end of the winter, a whole sack of very old potatoes will be heavily infected with invisible mould, especially if they are damp and have not been scrubbed. Dry, scrubbed potatoes are the best buy at this time of year.

FREEZE LEFTOVER FOOD AS SOON AS IT COOLS

If candida is stubborn, then leftover food could be keeping you ill, because when cooked food is kept at room temperature it becomes heavily infected with invisible moulds in less than an hour. Even ordinary refrigeration is not cold enough. Although the food looks and tastes all right, and does not upset other people, it can sometimes aggravate candida symptoms, causing bloating, wind and hot flushes in very sensitive people.

- Avoid using meat stock in vegetable soups—it ferments very rapidly indeed.
- Even vegetable soup ferments quickly, especially if it contains lentils or dried beans.
- Vegetables, especially root vegetables and green vegetables, are best eaten freshly cooked. You may find that they upset you almost as soon as they have cooled.

The above measures can sometimes bring very surprising improvements.

Some ways to freeze leftover food

Leftover roast meat can be sliced up and placed on a flat baking tray. Put empty plastic bags between the layers, cover the tray with another plastic bag and freeze it. You could prepare enough to last the week, and use it as needed.

Dried peas, beans and lentils can be cooked in the usual way, rinsed in cold water, frozen on a flat tray, then kept in plastic bags ready to use.

Rice and other cooked grains can be frozen in individual portions:

- Make a quantity and cool it straight away.
- Place individual portions in plastic containers.
- Stand them in the fast-freezing compartment of the freezer, then defrost them in a microwave oven as needed.

This information will help those who cannot take bread of any kind and who have to rely on cooked grains. It saves a lot of cooking time, especially if you need frequent snacks.

YOU CAN HEAL YOUR GUT

While the lining of the gut is in poor condition it will harbour candida. As natural healing progresses, nature will seal the gut and the mucous membranes throughout the body, so that candida eventually loosens its grip.

Remember to keep to the principles of the Hay diet

Fifty per cent raw vegetables and salads provide much of the raw material to do the job.

Extra virgin olive oil—at least 1–2 tablespoons per day— prevents yeasts from changing to their fungal form and helps to heal the gut. If your tongue is cracked and furred and your skin is dry, you may need much more oil—see chapter 13.
*Evening primrose oil—4–6 × 500 mg capsules per day—*is another powerful aid to healing mucous membranes. In Britain it is available on medical prescription for eczema and breast pain.

NATURAL TREATMENTS FOR CANDIDA

Lactobacillus acidophilus, the friendly bacteria

If you wait until you are fully on the anti-candida diet, and no longer taking sugar, yeast or alcohol, then you can replant the gut with friendly bacteria, which are available from health food shops in capsules. Lactobacillus acidophilus is an essential part of the treatment right from the beginning. You may be able to control candida with acidophilus alone if you take enough, provided you also keep strictly to the diet.

FRIENDLY BACTERIA

- They multiply in the gut, and fight candida for you.
- They help to control bloating and wind and to calm diarrhoea.
- They can firm the stools and add bulk to them.
- They can also help constipation.
- It may be some time before you feel the benefit of them.

Breaking the diet at this stage feeds the candida, making acidophilus ineffective.

Natural yoghurt also contains friendly bacteria, but many chronic candida sufferers are allergic to dairy products, yoghurt included.

How much acidophilus?
Two billion bacteria is the average effective dose in each capsule, but some brands contain far less, too little to be effective.

Acidophilus powder is much more expensive, but can be more effective than the capsules.
Refrigerate acidophilus and do not take it with hot food and drinks or the bacteria will die.

Vitamin and mineral supplements

If candida is severe you will need extra vitamins, minerals and evening primrose oil to strengthen immunity, repair the gut and mucous membrane, and increase energy levels. If you are very weak and deficient the supplement programme on p. 202 may help.

Herbal remedies

These can be highly effective. You would need to consult a medical herbalist.

ANTIFUNGAL TREATMENTS

If you are making steady progress on the diet and supplements you may not need further treatment. But if candida is stubborn and diet, acidophilus and vitamins do not entirely solve the problem, you may need an antifungal preparation as well. Unlike the short courses of treatment given for vaginal thrush, antifungal drugs and natural fungicides have to be taken continuously for up to three months.

Caprylic acid

This is a very powerful natural fungicide based on coconut. It can be highly effective, even in severe chronic candida. Ideally it should only be used under the professional supervision of a nutritional therapist, naturopath or a nutritionally orientated doctor. It is available without medical prescription from health food shops or directly from food supplement companies. For more information about the dose of caprylic acid see Erica White's *Beat Candida Cookbook*.

- Coconut is a common cause of allergic reactions.
- **No caprylic acid during pregnancy.**

Antifungal drugs

Antifungal drugs are readily available on medical prescription. Make sure you know what the side-effects are and keep a watch out for them.

NYSTATIN

This is generally considered to be the safest drug option. It comes as Nystan tablets or as a powder in a plastic carton, which can be much more effective. It is a fungal antibiotic, which is actually made from a fungus, and its effect can sometimes be dramatic when candida is overwhelming. However, it does occasionally cause reactions, including depression and bowel upsets.

Continue with the acidophilus

You need to take it in addition to any antifungal drugs or natural fungicides, so that there are friendly bacteria available to occupy the space left empty when candida dies.

- Remember that antifungal preparations do not kill friendly bacteria, they only kill yeasts and fungi. They are strictly a temporary help in cases where the infection is overwhelming.

So unless you also keep to the diet and work to strengthen your immune system at the same time so that the body can control candida by itself, candida may come rushing back whenever you try to reduce the medication.

DIE-OFF REACTIONS

When candida is starved by the diet and killed by antifungal preparations, dead candida and their toxins flood the system, and if the liver cannot keep up with the job of clearing them out, the usual symptoms may flare up again for a few days but should pass within a week or two.

- Always start with a very small dose of antifungal medication and increase it very gradually, to minimise die-off.
- If die-off is severe you may need to reduce the medication or stop it altogether until the symptoms clear.

CAUTION: If you are very severely affected by chronic candida, M.E. or chronic fatigue syndrome, it is inadvisable to take caprylic acid or any other natural antifungal medication or antifungal drugs without very expert help, because the build-up of toxins can overwhelm a debilitated liver and the die-off reaction could be severe enough to cause a relapse.

DIE-OFF OR ALLERGIC REACTION?
Unusual symptoms may indicate an allergic reaction to the treatment. Reactions to antifungal drugs are quite common.

CANDIDA AND MERCURY

If candida comes back every time you reduce the antifungal treatment, consider mercury sensitivity. Mercury from metal fillings mixes with the saliva and drips down into the gut, constantly killing the friendly bacteria. Having it removed could be a very short cut to recovery. Replacing amalgam fillings with white ones can be very expensive, but you can also spend a fortune on acidophilus and anti-candida medication over the years. In fact you could soon feel so much better without the mercury that you would be able to return to work. This has been my own experience (see p. 227).

KEITH'S STORY
Keith had two jobs and worked out several times a week at the gym. Always a heavy beer drinker, he began eating lots of sugar and chocolate in an effort to gain weight and improve his physique, seriously undermining his immunity over the years. Then when a 'flu virus came along he just could not fight it and

he never fully recovered. His GP conscientiously performed every possible test, and when they all came back negative he became so convinced Keith's symptoms were 'all in the mind' that he would not refer him to any other doctor or specialist.

Having been told that his illness was psychological, Keith tried to fight it with exercise, continuing to work out regularly, however hard it became. He felt endlessly tired and ill, but for the next ten years he soldiered desperately on for the sake of his young family. 'I just had to drink, my way of coping was to get a skinful.' He was still having his chocolate and three teaspoonfuls of sugar in his tea, believing he needed it for energy. He had persistent sore throats, chronic catarrh and dizzy spells. He had stomach pains and he felt so hot and burning all night that he hardly slept. He was underweight, full of worry and tension, and his hair was falling out.

Then one day he came across an article about M.E., and consulted a private medical specialist who diagnosed candida. He was on the right track at last. 'This diet is really tough. At first I felt I could never do it.' He was trying to change his diet and cope with a heavy job at the same time and it was making him very weak. Then he cut the sugar down too fast and lost his energy. He could not face the thought of going back to work next day but he knew his doctor would never sign him off sick. So he went to work and had a really bad day, but with high energy snacks and plenty of protein over the next few days he managed to recover.

After all that he changed his doctor. He found someone sympathetic to M.E., who signed him off work for several weeks to give him time to adapt to the diet and to recover his strength. His new GP also recommended a nutritional therapist and he keeps in close touch with her, too. Over the last three months he has put on weight, sleeps better, and his strength is returning at last. Now that he understands his illness he manages it very well indeed. His story demonstrates what illness is really like, that it seldom fits any diagnosis exactly.

CHAPTER 9

Are You Allergic?

Many of us are allergic without knowing it—I was myself. People with food intolerance frequently do not realise they are allergic at all unless they also suffer from well-recognised allergies like asthma or eczema. But allergic reactions are not confined to the air passages and skin, they occur right throughout the body, including the gut, and they can even affect the brain. So if you have migraine, arthritis, depression or irritable bowel, you could actually be as allergic as any asthmatic. Modern medicine persuades us to take drugs and medicines when we are ill, when in fact it often makes a lot more sense to take things away—in this case, to relieve the body of its burden of allergy.

Invisible symptoms

Seeing is believing to a medical mind. Eczema and asthma are readily detected, but most of the other symptoms of allergy are subjective, they are about the way we feel. They cannot be confirmed by laboratory testing so they go unrecognised and untreated. But chronic allergies of every kind can respond extremely well to nutritional medicine, beginning with the Hay diet. You may well obtain better results in the long term with diet than with drugs.

A surprising number of our everyday problems are associated with food intolerance, and once the offending foods are removed from the diet whole clusters of symptoms frequently disappear together. It has long been known that the same foods cannot possibly suit everybody. The ancient Egyptians very wisely considered that everybody's diet should be individually prescribed.

LOOK FOR FOOD INTOLERANCE IN THESE CONDITIONS

Migraine	Arthritis
Irritable bowel	Diarrhoea
Unexplained depression	Chronic fatigue
Overweight	Underweight
Nervous problems	Mental illness
Peptic ulcers	Low blood sugar
Eczema	Candida
Hyperactivity	Crohn's disease
Colitis	Hiatus hernia
M.E.	

This list is by no means complete!

If you can find no other reason for the symptoms listed over-leaf then you may be suffering from systemic reactions to common foods and additives. Symptoms appear gradually, after hours or even days, so the cause of the trouble is not recognised. The foods we eat most often, the ones we cannot do without, are most likely to cause trouble. Usually doctors can find nothing physically wrong.

Other symptoms include:

Low resistance to infection	Undue stress
Feeling constantly unwell	Low level of functioning
Frequent 'virus' infections	Frequent colds, mucus problems

But I could never give up my favourite food!
If you are allergic to any food and you continue to eat it, it will gradually undermine your health. You become increasingly tired and stressed, find it difficult to concentrate, and become

---

**THESE ARE COMMON SYMPTOMS OF
FOOD INTOLERANCE**

Pale, greyish complexion	Dark circles under the eyes
Compulsive eating	Poor appetite
Distension after meals	Mood swings
Low blood sugar	Undue fatigue
Rashes, eczema	Exhaustion
Drowsiness	Mental fogging
Mental tiredess	Aching limbs
Hyperactivity	Tension, anxiety
Depression	Migraine
Headaches	General sluggishness
Aggression	Muscle weakness
Irritable bowel	Irritable bladder
Nervous problems	Mental illness
Palpitations	Faintness
Crying spells	Urticaria (nettle rash)
General puffiness	Fluid retention
Conventional allergies	Joint pains

**Medical tests often prove negative
MOST OF THESE SYMPTOMS CAN BE
RELIEVED**

---

much more prone to infections. Going without it could give you a new lease of life, and many people find that after some time they can take a problem food now and again in moderation.

HOW CAN I TELL WHETHER I AM ALLERGIC TO FOOD?

The Hay diet is a simple elimination diet. If your allergy clears up on it, then you must have removed the offending food or additive. Most people can soon identify the culprit when they lapse back into bad habits!

THESE MOST COMMONLY CAUSE REACTIONS

Chemical additives	Colourings and flavourings
Chocolate	Sugar
White flour	White bread
Dairy products	Wheat and gluten
Citrus fruits	Pork, ham, bacon, sausages

Intolerance to natural foods

Any food can cause a reaction, but wheat and dairy products top the list. There is nothing wrong with these foods. They suit most people. They only upset those who have an allergic response to them.

ALLERGY CAN SLOW YOU DOWN

Many people cannot understand why they are constantly run down, often despite a healthy diet, or why they need so much more sleep and rest than everyone else. Certain foods and sometimes even inhaled allergens can exert powerful sedative effects on an allergic person. They can be as potent as alcohol or any drug, and over the years it can become increasingly difficult to function due to increasing tiredness and apathy.

People who appear dreamy, lazy, switched off, half-asleep,

or who suffer bouts of overwhelming drowsiness, can sometimes come to life in a surprising way once they find the cause of the trouble.

Do you wake up tired?

Is it difficult to get going in the mornings?
Do you wake late, midday perhaps?
Are you never punctual, despite your best intentions?
Are you always behind with your work?
Does tiredness limit your social life?
Are you sometimes drowsy when driving?
Do you fall asleep at awkward times during the day?
Do you hate letting people down over time?

You can dramatically increase your vitality!

- *Start with the Hay diet.*
  Processed foods can slow you down.
- *Avoid sugar and stimulants.*
- *Avoid foods to which you are intolerant:*
  Wheat and dairy products are very common causes of tiredness.
  Any other food to which you are intolerant can also sap your energy.

TREATING FOOD INTOLERANCE

Allergies are another expression of poor immunity, so by restoring natural immunity we can also reduce allergic sensitivity.

- Support the immune system with the Hay diet.
- Take vitamin and mineral supplements, too, if you are very debilitated (see the supplement programme on p. 202).
- Evening primrose oil is also quite powerfully anti-allergy.

Reduce the total load on the immune system

As well as cutting out any foods to which you are intolerant, remember that the mercury in dental fillings is a constant drain on the immune system.

Food combining can reduce allergic reactions

Remember also that when concentrated starch and concentrated protein are eaten together, the protein is not always sufficiently broken down, allowing large protein molecules such as histamine to be absorbed into the bloodstream and set up allergic reactions.

Candida frequently accompanies food intolerance

Many people with chronic candida have a 'leaky gut' which again allows large molecules of protein to leak into the bloodstream and set up allergic reactions to food.

Food intolerance and low blood sugar

When blood sugar levels are low, allergic sensitivity increases. Problem foods frequently cause blood sugar swings, and once they are removed from the diet, many people find that their blood sugar levels stabilise automatically. Others may improve to some extent, but the problem remains. Controlling blood sugar levels can reduce the severity of allergic reactions very considerably.

Do you lack essential oils?

If you have been following a low fat diet or if your diet is restricted, remember that substantially increasing your intake of natural oils can sometimes reduce allergic sensitivity to a remarkable degree.

FOOD INTOLERANCE IS A COMMON CAUSE OF DRUG DEPENDENCE

If your symptoms come rushing back every time you attempt to reduce your drugs, then the underlying problem has obviously not been identified and may well lie in your diet. When the symptoms of food intolerance are suppressed by drugs, food intolerances can multiply. Allergic people on long-term antidepressants, tranquillisers or steroids frequently suffer from multiple allergies requiring desensitisation. My own diet is still very restricted as a result.

DO I NEED TO BE DESENSITISED?

Possibly, if you cannot obtain a properly balanced diet because your range of safe foods is so limited, or if your diet is so restricted that you cannot maintain your normal body weight.

Does desensitisation work?
There is no guarantee. In my own case it gradually reduced the overall level of sensitivity and relieved many of the symptoms, but I was only able to widen my diet very slowly indeed over many years. Many people get much better results.

Food intolerance and mercury
If you have allergies and food intolerances which stubbornly persist despite treatment, suspect mercury sensitivity. Multiple metals in the mouth and multiple allergies frequently go together.

EPD (Enzyme Potentiated Desensitisation)

This is given by medical practitioners. It involves an intradermal injection into the skin, about every two to four months at the beginning. The injection contains a wide range of foods and/or inhaled allergens such as pollens, in homoeopathic dilution. The mixtures are the same for everyone. It also contains an enzyme thought to act directly on the immune system.

Be careful of taking megavitamins
EPD will work without the megadoses of vitamins A and D given to potentiate it. If treatments are frequent over a prolonged period of time they can sometimes build up to an overdose in the body, and the symptoms can be devastating. It happened to me, without warning: I felt marvellous for a while, too good to be true, and then it hit me very hard indeed.

IS YOUR DIET HIGH IN VITAMIN A?

- There are huge amounts of vitamin A in liver.
- Vitamins A and D are also present in most multivitamin tablets.

For further information on EPD, contact The National Society for Research into Allergy (see Useful Addresses).

Neutralising drops or injections

These are not the incremental allergy injections which were banned some years ago for safety reasons. These injections are self-administered, and the needle is so fine that they are practically painless. Dr John Mansfield uses this treatment and discusses it in his book *The Migraine Revolution*.

Action for M.E. produce a very helpful fact sheet comparing EPD and Neutralisation (see Useful Addresses).

ASTHMA? ECZEMA? HAY FEVER?

Make the food connection

What triggers your allergy? Is it pollen? Is it cow's milk? Is it stress? You may be surprised to know that the triggers are very often not the true causes at all. If you think of a gun, it will only fire if there is a bullet in it; remove the bullet and the trigger has no effect. Similarly, once you find the underlying cause of an allergy, the 'bullet' (which very often proves to be a food), then the stress or the pollen which triggered it may no longer affect you to the same extent. You may even find that the allergy clears up altogether.

Try the Hay diet first

Caroline's migraine struck her down whenever she ate dairy products, but to her great surprise she found that on the Hay diet she could take them without ill-effects. She felt better straight away—and the true culprits eventually proved to be sugar and white flour!

Brian's wheezing and hay fever no longer bothered him once he cut out dairy products.

Anne's eczema flared up under stress, but disappeared entirely once she gave up chocolate.

HELP FOR CHRONIC ASTHMA

More can be done for asthma than is generally realised, even by the medical profession. People who rely on drugs such as Becotide, Ventolin and even steroids all year round may be able to obtain substantial improvements and cut down on their drugs. Chronic asthma is seen not as a separate illness by itself, but as part of a much bigger picture, the tip of the iceberg.

Chronic asthma can respond very well indeed to the Hay diet
But be patient, it can take three to six months to feel the full benefit.

Keep your blood sugar level up

When blood sugar is normal, allergic reactions are less likely to happen. Wheezing in the night is often due to a drop in blood sugar levels. Not all of the foods involved in producing the total illness will result in asthma: they could produce any

---

CHRONIC ASTHMA—THE WHOLE PICTURE

Wheezing	Asthma attacks
Permanent sniff	Tiredness
Blocked nose	Irritability
Frequent colds	Nervousness
Chest infections	Emotional problems
Dry, itchy skin	Tension
Digestive upsets	Stomach aches
Joint pains	Poor immunity
Rashes	Eczema
Hay fever	'Virus' infections

These are systemic symptoms of allergy
They can be relieved

---

symptom at all. It could surprise you just how many of these problems can be relieved, and how quickly.

Drugs never cure asthma

They only control the wheezing for a day at a time, so if you continue taking foods which upset you, it will be a constant problem.

CAUTION! Keep on taking your drugs or inhalers

Make sure you are well established on the diet and feeling very much better before attempting to reduce the inhalers, otherwise the asthma will run out of control and the wheezing will come back, which can be dangerous. So reduce them very gradually indeed, and only under medical supervision.

WHICH FOODS MOST COMMONLY CAUSE WHEEZING?

CHILDREN	ADULTS
Eggs	Dairy products
Cow's milk	Wheat, yeast
Dairy products	Preservatives
Artificial colours	Coffee
Citrus fruits	Nuts, especially peanuts
Pork, bacon, ham, sausages	

Usually several different foods are involved in chronic asthma

Are you taking steroid drugs?

Anyone who has taken asthma drugs for a long time and who is severely debilitated may find they have multiple sensitivities to both foods and inhaled substances (see p. 139).

CAUTION: It is essential to consult a doctor who specialises in nutritional medicine if your problems are many and severe.
REPEAT WARNING: The sudden withdrawal of steroid drugs can be life-threatening.
Wait until you feel considerably better, then ask the doctor's advice. Keep yourself feeling reasonably well. Remember, the gentlest way to reduce any tablets is with a nail file.

Candida can be heavily involved in asthma, and it can be very severe, especially if you are taking steroid drugs.

Think seriously about mercury, too. Again, many people with this condition have a large number of metal fillings.

TESTING FOODS FOR ASTHMA? BE VERY CAREFUL INDEED!

If you are taking a suspect food in large amounts, cut it down very slowly to minimise discomfort from withdrawal symptoms. Once a food has been cut out for seven to ten days you become very much more sensitive to it when you first take it again.

Beware asthma attacks

Be extra careful, especially with children:

- Only try a very small amount of a suspect food to begin with, because you could get an asthma attack, even if you are just a chronic wheezer who rarely gets one.

What symptoms could I expect?
Remember that the food you are testing will not necessarily produce asthma and wheezing, it may produce another reaction altogether, commonly:

a 'cold', a sore throat, or a 'virus infection'.
nausea, vomiting: pork is a common culprit.
mood changes, hyperactivity.
rashes—any reaction at all.

Any other health problem you can solve will reduce the workload on the body, enabling it to cope very much more effectively with the asthma. If your asthma improves and you are sure which food is causing it, there is obviously no need to risk an attack by testing it.

Other causes of wheezing
Natural gas and calor gas fumes (see p. 150), also tobacco smoke.

ALLERGIES CAN MAKE YOUR HEART RACE

Dr Arthur Coca, a contemporary of Dr Hay, was an eminent American immunologist who made a very unscientific discovery. Dr Coca's wife was an invalid who was frequently rushed to hospital with severe attacks of palpitations, a fast-beating heart, but nothing was ever found to be wrong with her heart and no one could help her. Then one day she remarked to her husband that certain foods always made her heart beat faster, so Dr Coca began recording her pulse rate at regular intervals after she had eaten them. She then cut out the suspect foods and to their delight and amazement Mrs Coca got up and started living again. She was even able to dig the garden, and she lived to a healthy old age.

An excited Dr Coca presented his findings to his medical colleagues—but they froze him out, they fired him. They dismissed him as a simple quack, so he published, *The Pulse Test*, a little book written especially for patients, explaining how to use his method. It is still in print today.

ANNE'S STORY

Mrs Coca's story set Anne thinking. She had suffered frightening attacks of palpitations and faintness during the day for several months and no one knew why; at times she felt as if she would collapse. She worked very hard on the Hay diet, and once she had cut out all the processed foods she was able to see that these attacks were actually caused by the bananas she ate for breakfast every day.

Be very careful indeed when testing

If severe attacks like this do clear up on the Hay diet, be extra careful when you try any food you suspect of causing the trouble. The reaction could be very much more severe than it used to be, so try only a very little. Again, if you know for sure what has been upsetting you, then there is no real need to test it at all.

Allergic reactions can change
Be prepared for this, because having cut out a troublesome food for a while, you may find that it causes a different reaction altogether when you try it again.

WARNING Allergic reactions to food can sometimes be life-threatening. Devastating reactions like this are fortunately rare, and of course there is no substitute for medical treatment in an emergency.

GLUTEN-FREE, WHEAT-FREE, DAIRY-FREE MEALS

The simplest way to manage this diet is to have two cooked meals each day. It is quite easy to manage, whether you have a works canteen or are at home.

Protein meals are no problem. Just keep to plain home-cooked meat, fish or egg dishes with cooked vegetables or salad. Starch meals can be more of a challenge:

STARCH BREAKFASTS AND LIGHT LUNCHES
Millet flake porridge.
Muesli made with millet flakes.
Brown rice flake porridge.
Rice cakes topped with nut butter and sliced tomato.

Potato-based dishes
Leek and potato soup.
Sliced jacket potato with beans.
Jacket potato with vegetarian sauce.
Potato cake with salad.
Vegetarian shepherd's pie.
Vegetable hotpot.

Rice dishes
Rice mixed with vegetables.
Brown rice with ratatouille.

Brown rice with bean and vegetable stew.
Rice with vegetable curry.
Rice with stir-fried vegetables.
Rice and broad beans with vegetarian sauce.
Rice mixed with crunchy chopped raw vegetables and sun-
flower seeds.
Rice with sesame seed or cashew nut stir-fry.

The other gluten-free grains can be used instead of rice
Millet, buckwheat or quinoa

NO DAIRY FATS — NO MIGRAINE

Migraines regularly put Eileen in bed for twenty-four hours at
a time, and whenever she stopped the drugs the headaches
came back. For many years she resisted the idea of looking into
her diet, thinking that if the answer were that simple the doctor
would have known about it. Then, in an effort to slim, she
switched to skimmed milk and cut out the cheese—and she
was cured! The doctor was as surprised as she was.

ARTHRITIS? . . .

'The tests for arthritis are all negative, yet my foot is so
swollen I can't get my shoe on, and I can't even sleep for the
pain.' There is often a very simple answer to problems like
this, and this time it was tea and coffee! Two weeks later came
the report: 'I still can't believe it's that simple, but I haven't
had the tea or the coffee and I haven't had the swelling or the
pain. The effect was immediate, it's amazing.' Another person
with a similar problem recovered on the Hay diet plus the anti-
candida diet.

FIONA'S STORY

'People think she just can't be bothered, but I can see she is ill.'
Fiona's mother came looking for help. At the age of seventeen
her daughter was so tired that she had been forced to give up
her college studies. She was sleeping twelve or thirteen hours a

day, was difficult to rouse, and just sat all day in a stupor. It was difficult to get her to go out, and when she did go she just walked around like a zombie. She loved cheese sandwiches but had little appetite for anything else and she was definitely not having enough to eat. Would she consider changing her diet? 'Well, you don't think I want to be like this all my life, do you?' With her mother's dedicated help she cut out all dairy products and began the Hay diet with blood sugar control.

A great burden was lifted from Fiona in a very short time. She's not tired any more, she's enthusiastic and busy, she talks and she listens. Her confidence is growing and she is developing a really positive attiude to life. And she has even got a new job. She leaves home at 6.30 a.m. and returns at 6.30 p.m., yet she still has time to study for her 'A' level exams. Academically she has surprised everyone. She is happy on natural food now and the only thing she misses is her cheese roll—but after just a small amount of cheese on her salad, she promptly went back to being sleepy.

NO WHEAT − NO PROBLEM!
I feel so well now, so alert. I'm down to size fourteen from size eighteen, and I've been shopping! I've been overweight for such a long time, my legs were swollen, blown up like balloons, and my arms, I was puffed up everywhere. It started going down when I cut out wheat and everything with flour in it, and now I've cut down on the sugar and the salt as well. The salt pot was like the sugar pot to me! And my migraines have gone, too. The pain was awful, I used to lie in bed holding my head, but I don't need the tablets now. As long as I keep to the Hay diet I'm all right.

BORN TIRED!
I was born tired, I have been tired nearly all my life and I could never get enough sleep, not until I investigated my diet. Now I wake naturally at five or six in the morning, I cannot stay in bed. I need five or six hours' sleep now, instead of nine or ten,

and I could never have believed such a thing could happen. It's a new life.

ARE YOU SENSITIVE TO NATURAL GAS?

Did you know about indoor air pollution?

People who are affected by natural gas seldom realise it. It can make you very tired and irritable, especially at mealtimes when the gas cooker is on. It can also make you very tired and sleepy in the evenings when the house is full of fumes, especially if you also use a gas fire. Suspect it if you cannot smell gas at all, or if you can detect the slightest trace of it when other people cannot.

Petrol fumes and natural gas are related

They are both petrochemicals. So if you suffer from nausea or from any other symptoms while travelling by car it may be worth turning the gas off at the stopcock for 24 to 48 hours and ventilating the house, to see if you feel better. Gas central heating alone will probably not affect you, as the fumes are sucked straight outside, but if you are very severely affected you could try spending a holiday in an all-electric household.

Oil-fired central heating and bottled gas can have similar effects.
The fumes from indoor painting and decorating can also sometimes make an allergic person feel depressed, exhausted and ill.

CHAPTER 10

The Allergic Child

Allergy is becoming more and more common amongst children. Bottle-feeding and the early introduction of solid food increase the risk. If a child has many health problems, if he is unhappy and failing to thrive, yet doctors cannot help, it may be worth investigating his diet. Allergic children are frequently born to allergic parents, people with a history of hyperactivity, migraine or unexplained depression and nervous problems, as well as conventional allergies like asthma and eczema. However, they do also turn up unexpectedly in other families.

These delicate children can be difficult to manage because they never feel really well. They often get pathetically upset over small things. Mood swings from extreme anger to prolonged crying are common. They may fight and bicker constantly and many are impossible at home. Often just a change to natural whole food brings a surprising improvement, enough to really open your mind to the food connection. A change to wholemeal bread may well be enough to calm a child considerably.

The pain of watching a child's health deteriorate and finding no one in the medical profession who can help is still a common experience for many parents. Usually nothing is found to be physically wrong, and most of the symptoms clear up once the offending foods are removed.

THE ALLERGIC CHILD

Lack of confidence
Behaviour problems
Nightmares
Nervousness
Headaches, migraine
Poor resistance to infection
Loss of weight
Always thirsty
Depression
Panic attacks
Loose stools
Physical inco-ordination
Accident-prone
Excessive sweating
Abdominal distension
Dry, itchy skin
Hyperactivity or
  overactivity
Stomach ache
Letter reversal
Insecurity (not happy away
  from his parents)

Extreme emotional
  sensitivity
Mood swings
Aggression
Persistent tiredness
Frequent 'virus'
  infections
Itchy nose
Loss of appetite
Listlessness
Bedwetting
Tension
Constipation
Clumsy
Always falling over
Nausea and sickness
Rashes
Feeling extra cold
Slow and dreamy
Constantly aching legs
Fits associated with
  migraine

A lovely child can usually be seen underneath
all this misery
**MOST OF THESE SYMPTOMS CAN
BE RELIEVED**

Why is allergy so much more common in children these days?

- Because we are largely unaware of the part food can play in allergy.
- Because too much junk food and soft drinks weaken a child's immunity.
- Mercury crosses the placental barrier and affects the foetus, and I do wonder how much this, too, is lowering our children's immunity, especially since in Britain, until recently, many mothers took advantage of the offer of free dental treatment during pregnancy. Nowadays in Britain, as a precaution, mercury amalgam is not recommended to be inserted or removed during pregnancy.

An allergic child is better off without mercury amalgam
White fillings are obviously better.

ALLERGIC TENSION-FATIGUE

These children are always tired, pale and irritable, often with great dark circles under their eyes and a grey, toxic complexion. They can be extremely tense, fidgety and demanding. Many dislike being left alone, have great difficulty getting to sleep, and may have frequent nightmares. They suffer greatly from stress and can be pathetically sensitive. Amazingly, such children can blossom into relaxed and happy confidence once the allergic source of their illness is identified and the offending foods are removed.

LEARNING PROBLEMS

Allergic children are often under-achievers, with poor concentration and great difficulty in learning to read and write, even despite an obviously bright mind. Letter reversal problems are common. But they can very quickly realise their potential once they are well.

LOW RESISTANCE TO INFECTION

Life for many allergic children is one long round of infections and antibiotics, and they become more debilitated all the time. Their system may eventually become so overburdened with allergy that it cannot cope with infection at all. Suspect food intolerance in any child who suffers this way. Cow's milk is the commonest cause, but other foods can be involved as well.

'Colds' and 'viruses'

Many allergic children have mucus problems: a permanent and irritating sniff, an itchy nose, sneezing and frequent colds. Recurrent sore throats, huge tonsils and attacks of tonsillitis can equally be due to allergy. Again, once the offending foods are removed the infections gradually decrease in frequency and severity and the tonsils gradually reduce in size.

Restoring natural immunity

Repeated antibiotics weaken our immunity, because if the body is never allowed to fight its own battles, the immune system gradually becomes less efficient. The way forward is to gradually strengthen natural resistance with natural food, avoiding processed foods and removing any foods to which the child is intolerant. As natural resistance improves, the infections become less severe and less frequent, until antibiotics are no longer required, then eventually they clear up altogether. Extra vitamins and minerals and evening primrose oil will help to speed recovery.

Enzyme Potentiated Desensitisation (EPD) can also be very helpful to a child over three years old with devastatingly low immunity, eczema, asthma or any other allergic condition. In desperate cases it can be given to children under three years.

EVENING PRIMROSE OIL AND ALLERGY

Many allergic children have an enzyme deficiency, which means they cannot absorb essential oils from their food, and their health can sometimes improve quite dramatically on a supplement of evening primrose oil. It is anti-allergy, mentally calming, and it can improve dry skin quite amazingly. Some hyperactive children have been known to settle down completely on high doses of evening primrose oil, and may even begin to tolerate foods which had previously been a problem to them.

Shirley Flack discusses this further in her book *Hyperactive Children*. She also gives some very encouraging case histories of recovered children.

Taking evening primrose oil

If there is a reaction to it or if it has no effect by mouth the end of the capsule can be cut off and the oil can be rubbed into the skin.

WARNING: Children who have temporal lobe epilepsy should not take evening primrose oil except under medical supervision.

Essential oils are also essential for normal growth. Breast milk is very high in essential fats, and low in protein, yet babies grow at an amazing rate.

THE ALLERGIC CHILD'S DIET

Be very careful indeed

Children's diets can be extremely difficult to manage, especially if there are several problem foods. The smaller the child, the more careful you have to be to keep her feeling as well as possible. Elimination dieting can be physically and

---

WHICH FOODS UPSET ALLERGIC CHILDREN MOST OFTEN?

Sugar	White flour
Artificial colourings	Monosodium glutamate
Soft drinks, especially cola	Food additives of all kinds
Wheat	Citrus fruits
Pork, bacon, ham	Fish
Dairy products	Tap water
Sugary breakfast cereals	Sausages, especially frankfurters

All other highly processed foods

---

psychologically devastating to a child. It is easier to withdraw one type of food at a time, and to let her get used to being without it before withdrawing anything else.

Withdrawal symptoms can sometimes be severe

The child may suffer severe food cravings or stomach pains, for example.

- Withdraw foods very slowly and always substitute something equally nutritious which she enjoys.
- Watch her weight *very* carefully indeed.
- Immune support is essential: extra vitamins and evening primrose oil. Biocare supply vitamin and mineral capsules specifically designed for hyperactive and allergic children. See Useful Addresses.

MILK ADDICTION
This is not uncommon in babies who are intolerant of milk. Often they are fretful and colicky, and they may become so addicted to milk that they want nothing else. They can be very

difficult to feed with solid food, and very reluctant to give up their bottle feeds as they grow older. Milk is also a common cause of hyperactivity and underactivity.

WHAT ABOUT CALCIUM?
Sugar and sweetened foods all rob us of calcium, as do tea and coffee and too much salt. But there is plenty of calcium in natural food of all kinds, including:

- Green leafy vegetables and whole grains.
- Eggs, nuts, seeds and beans.
- Fish like salmon and sardines which have edible bones.

You will need professional help with the diet
Dietitians can help with intolerance to dairy products, but they may not be accustomed to treating other food intolerances. A nutritional therapist would be able to help.

Are You Allergic? by Dr William Crook is extremely helpful to the parents of allergic children, but it is long out of print. You may be able to obtain it through public libraries.

HYPERACTIVE CHILDREN

Being lighter in weight, children react to chemical ingredients in foods more strongly than adults, because they get a bigger dose in relation to their size. And not only severely hyperactive children are affected by additives and processed foods. Any child who tends to get upset more than you feel is normal could become considerably calmer and more reasonable on a more natural diet.

Most hyperactive children are allergic

Many will fit somewhere into the picture of the allergic child given above. If a natural diet without additives and processed food does not entirely solve the problem, suspect dairy

---

SOME SYMPTOMS OF HYPERACTIVITY

Overactive	Nervous, excitable
Impulsive	Demanding
Impatient	Easily frustrated
Explosive	Temper tantrums
Mood swings	Aggressive
Unreasonable behaviour	Violent
'As if driven by a motor'	Sleeplessness
Rages	Disruptive behaviour
Anti-social	Anti-everything
Cries easily	Clumsy, unco-ordinated
Uncooperative	Totally negative, impossible

Overactive or hyperactive?
A diet of natural food will calm any child

---

products and the gluten grains, especially wheat. Any food can cause hyperactivity, but those in the box on p. 156 are the most likely. *The Hyperactive Child* by Belinda Barnes and Irene Colqhoun is a very great help.

UNDERACTIVE CHILDREN

Children who are passive, who are too quiet, nervous and withdrawn are as typically allergic as hyperactive children, but because they are not disruptive, because they are 'too good', their plight is overlooked. Their allergies slow them down, often making them dreamy and mentally fogged. They are exceptionally shy, and often cannot bear to be separated from their parents, and may be school refusers. Later on they may become isolated and bullied at school, and school attendance may be poor because they suffer such frequent infections. But they can come to life and change out of all recognition once the burden of allergic illness is lifted and they feel well again.

ALLERGIC REACTIONS CAN CHANGE

Childhood allergies like asthma and eczema often clear up as we grow older, but unless we are familiar with the pattern of allergic illness we may not realise that we could in fact still be allergic. An asthmatic child who grows out of the asthma but then develops migraine, nervous problems or joint pains, would not usually connect these with allergy, and nor would the doctor.

The homoeopathic view of how illness develops is highly relevant to allergy. Here is what can happen in a child intolerant to cow's milk:

1 Colic as a baby.
2 Frequent infections as a young child.
3 Eczema.
4 Persistent cough.
5 Wheezing.
6 Asthma.
7 Nervous and emotional problems, shyness.

Remember that infections and allergies are both expressions of poor immunity. Colic is often due to cow's milk. A breast-fed baby will sometimes react to cow's milk in its mother's diet.

The homoeopathic theory

A baby with colic and frequent infections, for example, will often go on to develop a predictable sequence of other problems. Again, the main cause of this chain of events is frequently cow's milk and the other dairy products.

- If the underlying allergic cause of the colic and poor immunity is not immediately identified and dealt with, the illness goes deeper.
- Eczema then develops, still a relatively superficial problem.
- Again, if the cause of the eczema is still not dealt with at source, if the offending food is not removed from the diet, the damage goes deeper still, causing cough, wheezing, chest infections and eventually asthma.
- The next and deepest level of allergy is the brain, and that is when nervous symptoms appear.

CHILDHOOD ASTHMA

Early warning signs of asthma before the wheezing appears

- Sensitivity to wind and cold air.
- Frequent colds and chest infections.
- A dry or tickling cough at night which no cough medicines ever help.
- Coughing after exercise.

Again, the underlying problem is very often an intolerance to cow's milk.

Medical treatment for asthma does not deal with the causes

Neglect of the true causes from early childhood accounts for much of the huge rise in asthma. Medical treatment is superficial, it just relieves the symptoms. Drugs and inhalers have only a temporary effect on the wheezing. Becotide works in a different way but the symptoms usually come back if you stop it altogether. The market for asthma drugs is therefore bottomless, and allergic illness continues.

To prevent the asthma running out of control, do not stop taking inhalers or any other medical treatment until a child is well enough to do without them. They can then be reduced very gradually under medical supervision.
Read: *Asthma Epidemic* by Dr John Mansfield.

PETS AND ASTHMA

Pets, especially cats, dogs and birds, are among the commonest causes of asthma in children. Animal dander is composed of microscopic particles of skin which settle on carpets, furniture and curtains and accumulate in the air. This is what can irritate eyes, nose and lungs. It also contributes to coughs, colds, chest infections and general debility. If a child has eczema, asthma, food intolerance or any other allergy, it is wise not to have a bird or animal in the house.

If, when you first get your pet, your child's eyes or nose run or he becomes obviously unwell, it may be better to part with it straight away if you can. Some children are so sensitive that they will never be really well while there is a pet in the house. But exposure to a pet will not always produce symptoms straight away, depending on how sensitive the child is. He may become unwell over weeks or months, so you may not realise that the pet is responsible.

If you already have a pet and your child has asthma it is sure to be a major cause of trouble. If you keep it out of the child's bedroom, hoover frequently and ventilate the house every day, opening all the doors and windows to get rid of the dander in the air, it could result in considerable improvement. If you are seriously considering parting with your pet, note whether there is an improvement when you go on holiday, or get the pet looked after for a couple of weeks.

House dust control

A child may spend twelve hours out of twenty-four in his bedroom, so it is worth paying attention to the dust there.

Desensitisation

If you cannot part with your pet and, despite dieting and house dust control, asthma is still a problem, Enzyme Potentiated Desensitisation can sometimes help.

WHO CAN HELP AN ALLERGIC CHILD?

The Department of Immunology in any large hospital
You would need an immunologist or a paediatric allergist.

Doctors who specialise in allergy and nutritional medicine.
These are usually private but you can sometimes be referred to them by the GP on the NHS. See Useful Addresses.

Naturopaths and nutritional therapists
These specialists can help with the diagnosis and treatment of food intolerance.

The Hyperactive Children's Support Group
This charitable organisation helps hyperactive and allergic children and their parents. They also produce an extremely helpful journal.

The National Society for Research into Allergy
The society has information on Enzyme Potentiated Desensitisation (EPD). See Useful Addresses.

CHAPTER 11

Help for M.E.

There is an alarming increase in severe and disabling chronic fatigue and M.E. (myalgic encephalomyelitis). People of all ages, young children included, are lying at home in bed for long periods of time, many so weak and lifeless that they can hardly lift a finger. Fifty years ago M.E. was almost unheard of—we are witnessing the advance of yet another new illness. This devastating neurological condition is often associated with a virus infection or candida, and sometimes with mercury toxicity.

The tragedy is that most people, including the medical profession, still believe that there is no effective treatment for M.E., because they know little of the powerful alternatives which exist in complementary medicine. Most journalists are equally unaware. Yet many people can be substantially relieved if they are willing to change their diet.

Is it really M.E. at all?

M.E. is a complex condition involving a great many different factors, and they vary from person to person. Most people who believe they may have M.E. are actually suffering from chronic fatigue. This is severe and prolonged fatigue, accompanied by a long list of other symptoms for which no cause can be found. And it is generally much easier to treat because victims of chronic fatigue do not usually have the devastating muscle fatigue and profound physical and mental exhaustion so typical of M.E.

Early diagnosis is vital

If you have severe muscle problems and you suspect M.E., remember that there are other conditions to be considered and excluded before the diagnosis is made, so make sure you get a thorough physical check-up.

Find a doctor who accepts M.E. and can make the diagnosis

Make this an absolute priority so that you can be signed off straight away from work, college or school, because immediate rest is vital to prevent you from getting any worse. Never overexert yourself. Some people have been known to become more disabled by their failure to rest and accept limitations, so conserve your energy. Learning to pace yourself is the key to a better quality of life.

MUSCLE WEAKNESS

Few people understand the level of disability M.E. can cause. You may have difficulty walking, climbing stairs or even standing for any length of time. Ordinary housework becomes a major undertaking. Cleaning, using the vacuum cleaner and even bed-making can be exhausting. Peeling vegetables can take forever. Muscles may sometimes become so weak and painful that it is impossible to dress, comb your hair, write or even use a knife and fork.

All these can play a part

- An unnatural or unbalanced diet.
- Too little concentrated protein—it builds muscle.
- Very low blood sugar: too little concentrated starch in the diet can lead to depleted starch reserves in the muscles.
- Food intolerance, especially to wheat and gluten.

164

M.E.—MYALGIC ENCEPHALOMYELITIS
A HUMAN 'POWER FAILURE'

It can follow:
'Flu, glandular fever, vaccination
A virus attack or gastro-enteritis

**Muscle fatigue
is the distinguishing feature of M.E.**
Muscle twitching and spasm
Weak, sore, tender muscles with constant pain
Intense and overwhelming physical exhaustion
triggered by trivial exercise

Devastating mental exhaustion
Poor concentration, poor short-term memory
Difficulty focusing, blurred vision
Even reading can prove too much

THIS IS A RELAPSING ILLNESS
Other symptoms include:
Alcohol intolerance
All the symptoms of a chronic infection
A long list of unexplained symptoms

- Remember also that candida can sometimes contribute to muscle pain and tenderness.
- Removing mercury can sometimes improve muscle tone very considerably. Just one filling may prove to be a serious health hazard.

BEAT BACKACHE
My back never stopped aching, the vertebrae were constantly slipping out of line. I could hardly stand, and for several years

the pain and exhaustion forced me to lie down several times throughout the day, yet doctors could find nothing wrong. The Hay diet and blood sugar control worked wonders, as did cutting out wheat and gluten. My muscle-tone improved, the vertebrae stayed put and the pain began to fade. Finally, removing mercury and all the other metal from my teeth has strengthened me and my muscles beyond belief.

YOU CAN HELP TO CONTROL RELAPSES WITH DIET

The Hay diet is a powerful weapon in the fight against M.E. By keeping your diet absolutely natural and absolutely right in every respect you can learn to control more of the fluctuations in the way you feel.

All these can contribute to a relapse:

- Too drastic a change in diet—change it slowly.
- Allowing blood sugar levels to drop too low.
- Incompatible mixtures of food.
- Allergic reactions to natural foods.
- A flare-up of candida.

Minor stresses of all kinds can upset a sick person much more severely than they would normally.

Keep to the Hay diet

It is absolutely essential to keep to safe, natural food and never to take sugar, processed food or soft drinks of any kind while you are as ill as this. When you are so weak it does not take much to knock you down. Pure fruit juices, fresh fruit and salad can do much to revive you.

166

CHRONIC HYPOGLYCAEMIA AND M.E.

M.E. victims often suffer from devastating hypoglycaemia

These symptoms are common to both:

Exhaustion	Forgetfulness
Depression	Allergies
Headaches	Lack of co-ordination
Irritability	Muscle weakness
Dizziness	Numbness, cramps
Mental confusion	Muscle-twitching
Sweating	Difficulty keeping warm
Difficulty focusing	Fainting, blackouts

**MERCURY, TOO, CAN CAUSE
SYMPTOMS LIKE THESE**

M.E. AND CHRONIC FATIGUE SYNDROME ARE
IMMUNE DISORDERS

Viruses are everywhere, but we only fall victim to them when our resistance is low, when our immune defences are not working properly. The immune system is spread right throughout the body—every tissue and every organ has its own defence system. A tendency to poor immunity can also be inherited: M.E. sufferers often find that their children have a tendency to similar problems. Remember that allergies, too, are an expression of poor immunity.

All these can weaken our immunity over the years:

- An unbalanced diet.
- Too much heavily processed food.

- Too much alcohol.
- Years of stress, overwork and fatigue
- Chronic hypoglycaemia
- Undiagnosed food allergies
- Chronic candida
- Powerful drugs taken long term

And remember: mercury is a constant drain on the immune system
M.E. can sometimes be substantially relieved by removing mercury and all the other metals from the mouth.

Virus or fungus?

It would not be surprising if the initial 'virus' attack in M.E. were actually an acute attack of candida, especially since candida is not medically recognised. Many M.E. victims with chronic 'flu symptoms have failed to consider candida seriously enough. It is much more common in M.E. than we realise and it can sometimes be very difficult indeed to recognise, even for an experienced nutritional therapist.

Virus AND fungus?

Even when it has been confirmed that you have a virus infection, you could actually also have a fungal infection. Since candida is more treatable, it could be worth trying the anti-candida diet if your progress is slow.

A MEDICAL MYSTERY — PETER'S STORY
I've been ill for five years. The first three years were terrible: I had terrifying blackouts with five admissions to the intensive care unit in one year. They tested me for absolutely everything but even then I got no diagnosis. It was demoralising to be told there was nothing wrong, it made me feel worse than ever. Apparently no one dared suggest M.E. because they had no

effective treatment to offer, but it was worse not knowing. Eventually I gave up on the medical profession, I just listened to my body and I began to get better.

The blackouts always came after sweet foods and a couple of drinks. I would wake in the night feeling hot, uncomfortable and ill; I would go to get a drink and the next thing I knew my wife was trying to revive me. But the last time I had no warning at all, and I was so pale and so still that my wife thought I must have died. That's when I stopped drinking alcohol and I haven't had a blackout since.

Some people did suggest that I try alternative medicine but I thought I was much too ill for such simple remedies. I felt so terrible, and the things that were happening to me were so dramatic that I just couldn't believe that diet and vitamins could possibly be powerful enough to help; I didn't want to get involved. But now I'm on a completely natural diet and I've cut out dairy products—I feel so much better without them. I've also cut out sugar and caffeine and I've cut the salt right down, too.

First to disappear were the chest pains—they were keeping me awake for an hour every night. I still have aches and pains and I can still get restless at night, but everything is improving. I'm taking vitamin and mineral supplements, too, and now, within three months, there is colour in my cheeks and my energy is beginning to come back. Consulting a nutritional therapist was the best thing I ever did.

CHAPTER 12

Not All in the Mind

People with long-standing nervous and emotional problems, for which no cause can be found, commonly also have an assortment of physical problems which are all too often dismissed as 'all in the mind'. Conventional medicine and psychiatry are of limited help to many of us because they treat the mind alone. Consequently there are thousands of us whose problems persist, despite every effort to help. By contrast, complementary medicine treats the whole person, mind and body together, and when mental and physical problems are treated together they clear up together.

Internal stress

The idea that stress can be caused internally—biochemically—is unfamiliar to most of us, although Freud himself predicted it many years ago. Food frequently causes more stress than environmental factors, and that makes it a lot easier to control than many of the other stresses we encounter. Remove the stress in your diet, and external pressures become very much easier to handle. Nutritional treatment can often work faster and more effectively than drugs for everyday problems like this.

But how can changing my diet possibly help my mind?
Most people, doctors among them, tend to assume that the mind works independently of the body. But every organ of the body, the brain included, is entirely constructed and maintained by molecules derived from the food we eat; so by improving the quality of our food we can substantially improve our state of mind, often in a surprisingly short time.

170

The brain is a complex mass of nervous tissue made up largely of water and fats, especially the essential fatty acids found in the natural oils so seriously lacking in our diet today. It depends on a rich supply of vitamins and minerals and a steady and even supply of glucose. It needs amino acids (protein), too—in fact it demands supernutrition if we are to get the best out of it.

A nervous person needs a natural diet

People with mental or nervous problems may well be consuming large amounts of convenience food. Many of us cannot handle so much of it, or in fact cope with it at all. We require an absolutely all-natural diet; we have no alternative if we are ever to function properly. A new diet is a small price to pay for a new life.

THIS IS AN UNHEALTHY STATE OF MIND
It can be reversed!

Forgetful	Moody
Dreamy	Easily confused
Easily stressed	Irritable
Depressed	Apathetic
Impatient	Bored
Fearful	Angry
Mentally tired	Negative
Poor concentration	Bad dreams
Sleeping problems	Anxious
Panicky	Shy

THE BRAIN IS THE FIRST TO RESPOND
TO A NATURAL DIET

- Preservatives, added to prevent food spoiling, slow biological activity. and can therefore slow our own mental and physical activity.
- Toxicity from too much highly processed food has a similar effect.

The chemical balance of the mind depends first of all on the balance of our diet and on the balance of each individual food within it, and when vital vitamins and minerals are processed out of food its natural balance is destroyed. The Hay diet improves your state of mind because it consists of the whole, balanced foods the human body is naturally designed to handle, which it can use to restore and maintain its natural equilibrium.

ADRENALINE AND YOU

Despite our ignorance of its needs, the body struggles valiantly to keep us on an even keel; the symptoms of stress are caused by its efforts to help, they are a signal to us that something is wrong.

- Fear and emotional distress cause a flow of adrenaline, which overstimulates the system, producing the symptoms of stress.
- Sugar and stimulants have similar effects, resulting in additional surges of adrenaline.
- Any food to which you are intolerant will also cause the adrenaline to flow. Remember that allergic conditions like asthma and eczema are commonly associated with nervous problems.

Stabilising blood sugar levels by adjusting the diet can therefore reduce the overall level of anxiety. Strict blood sugar control is the key to effective stress management.

PANIC ATTACK? OR HYPO ATTACK?

A mix of diet and emotions

A surge of adrenaline can produce
Anxiety, tension, nervousness
Fear, panic attacks
Nausea, sweating
A racing heart
Fainting, blackouts

**SUGAR AND STIMULANTS
FURTHER STIMULATE
THE ADRENAL GLANDS**
**causing more adrenaline to flow
at a time when we are already flooded with it!**

All this effort on the part of the body can drain us, leaving us weak and exhausted for a long time afterwards. We can therefore help ourselves tremendously by knowing which foods and drinks to avoid so that adrenaline is kept to a minimum.

An empty stomach can aggravate nervous symptoms
Remember that the brain cannot store glucose, so when the blood sugar falls after some time without food, adrenaline is produced to release stored glucose from the liver. But the adrenaline can also produce nervous symptoms at the same time. You can avoid this surge of adrenaline by eating regular meals with snacks in between if necessary, to keep blood sugar levels steady.

Make sure you get enough to eat during the day

Insufficient food, especially inadequate amounts of complex carbohydrate foods like wholemeal bread and potatoes, can keep blood sugar levels persistently low despite an all-natural diet, and keep our nerves constantly on edge despite frequent snacking. You will be surprised how much calmer you feel once you are eating more.

Are you drinking enough water?

Just drinking more water every day can be surprisingly helpful in clearing your head and reviving you generally. If you are very dehydrated you may not feel the benefit for several days.

But I have nervous problems despite a healthy diet

Are you allergic? If the Hay diet with blood sugar control does not solve the problem, you could also be suffering from intolerance to certain foods—remember that they can cause blood sugar swings just as stimulants do. In most cases blood sugar levels return to normal once they are identified and removed from the diet. Common problems like asthma, eczema, migraine and irritable bowel frequently accompany nervous symptoms. So do many other physical problems not normally associated with allergy or food intolerance.

BRAIN ALLERGIES
Brain allergies are extremely common but rarely recognised. Any food can be responsible, but suspect those you eat often:

- Dairy products can turn some of us into nervous wrecks.
- Wheat is an amazingly common cause of depression.
- Fish can sometimes have a devastating effect on mood, especially as sea fish contains mercury.

Not All in the Mind by the late Dr Richard McKarness, psychiatrist, will open your eyes to the magnitude of this problem in a very readable way.

Mercury targets the brain and nervous system

People with unexplained nervous and emotional problems often obtain substantial relief by changing their diet, but the improvement may still not be all they had hoped. Getting rid of mercury can solve many more problems (see chapter 16).

Before you forget how things used to be . . .
Write down the symptoms before you begin changing your diet—all of them, mental and physical (the list could be very long)—then cross them off as they evaporate. It will encourage you enormously.

A NIGHTMARE DIET?
Not at all! All you have to do is change your cookbooks. There are lots of recipe books written by people with similar problems and they all live very well, if a little differently. Just keep strictly to the rules until you have recovered, then you will learn what compromises you can make, if any.

BEAT SHYNESS

Most people would not see this as a health problem at all. They just get on with life as best they can, believing it to be an unfortunate aspect of their character. But the World Health Organisation defines good health as 'a state of complete mental, physical and *social* well-being' and a very shy person is rarely physically fit. How would you rate your level of fitness on a scale from one to ten? Shyness is just one part of an overall problem.

Won't I grow out of it?

To a certain extent perhaps, but there is absolutely no need to wait: you could experience considerable relief in a very short time, starting with the Hay diet and blood sugar control. If you have always been shy you will find it hard to believe it can be relieved at all, let alone by such simple measures. Most of us experience occasional shyness, but for some of us it can interfere with life in a big way.

WHY BE SHY?

How do you feel about . . .

using the telephone?	answering the doorbell?
asking for things in shops?	speaking up in class?
meetings, parties?	talking to strangers?
making conversation generally?	showing affection?
expressing your true feelings?	saying NO?

ALL THESE CAN BE RELIEVED!

Are you frequently and unnaturally afraid?

- Are you mysteriously embarrassed and self-conscious in the company of all but family and close friends?
- Despite a bright and original mind, have you nothing much to say?
- Do you keep quiet for fear of saying the wrong thing and making a fool of yourself?
- Do you avoid parties and social gatherings?
- Have you little interest in your appearance?
- Do you retreat to the safety of your room, alone with the TV or computer?
- Is your self-esteem at rock bottom?
- Is it difficult to cope with everyday life?

Don't die of loneliness!

You will be very surprised at just how much all this can be relieved, and how quickly. Holistic anxiety management works very well for most of us once the food connection has been made. You could be delighted to find that problems you always believed to be part of you prove to be nothing more than the symptoms of an unsuitable diet—and that they promptly disappear once it is put right.

————— *HAVE YOU EVER SUFFERED FROM . . .* —————

colic as a baby?
eczema, rashes?
wheezing, asthma, hay fever?
poor immunity, frequent colds?

Do you sleep late?
Is it hard to wake up? Does it take a long time?
Do you wake up tired and irritable?
Are you somewhat disorganised? Do you live in a muddle?
This picture will be familiar to many a shy and nervous person, and again the underlying cause is very often just an unsuitable diet:

- too little fresh fruit and salad
- no natural vegetable oils
- low blood sugar
- an intolerance to processed food in general
- possibly also an intolerance to dairy products or wheat

**REMEMBER THAT ONE IN TEN OF US
NEEDS SUPERNUTRITION**
if we are ever to function properly
It may enable you to beat the rest!

As you build yourself up physically, on the Hay diet and the supplement programme on p. 202, and as your body chemistry gradually comes back into balance, you may well find that your shyness is not quite such an integral part of you after all. Inhibitions evaporate and you begin to relax in the company of other people. Motivation and concentration also improve, and you become much more productive. Then, as it becomes easier to cope, your confidence grows and a stronger, more liberated personality begins to emerge. Who knows, you may even come to appreciate yourself—it can work wonders for your self-esteem!

Allergies and nervous problems often run in families
Sometimes there is a family history of allergies, food intolerance or coeliac disease.

Change your diet slowly

The anxiety may well get worse for a time initially, especially if you have been having lots of sweet foods or soft drinks, particularly cola, or drinking milk in large quantities. The remedy is to keep your blood sugar level steady with plenty of natural carbohydrate foods. If you are drinking a lot of milk, this may be contributing to the problem.

COME OUT OF YOUR SHELL!
Like the hermit crab, you could very soon leave it behind. People begin to catch glimpses of the real you, and you could soon find yourself talking to people quite naturally. I could never be myself, I was always an onlooker, longing to join in. I could never show affection, never speak my mind, and I'm still shy at times, but since working on my diet I have changed almost out of recognition.

Shyness can be disabling

Many of us, often highly talented people who have much to offer, find ourselves mysteriously shy and lacking in confidence. Everyday situations can eventually become so stressful that we find ourselves struggling to hold down a job or unable to face employment at all. This situation is becoming increasingly common, even amongst school-leavers. Many a young person who struggled through school is devastated to find that he or she cannot face work at all.

Faced with the threat of losing your job or your place at college or university?
Just work hard on your diet and lifestyle in every possible way, and you will be surprised at how fast things can improve. Hidden talents emerge, and you begin to discover your true potential. Young people in particular can respond very quickly indeed to improvements in diet.

What are your favourite foods?

- Do you have milk and cheese every day?
- Do you eat white bread, white pasta or white rice daily?
- Do pizzas, pies and pot noodles make up a large part of your diet?
- Do you crave sweet things?
- Do you eat sweets and chocolate every day?
- Do you have biscuits or cake every day?
- Do you consume large quantities of soft drinks?

What about the foods you are *not* eating!

Once again the essential oils really are essential!
Drastically increase fresh fruit and salad, substitute it for unhealthy snacks. Eat plenty of vegetables, cooked and raw.

Take extra care of yourself!
If you have struggled with your nerves at school, be extra care-ful with your diet when you leave home to study or to work, because without a good supply of fresh fruit and salad, and at least one substantial hot meal with meat and vegetables every day, you could find yourself in trouble. Motivation and concen-tration can be seriously impaired by a poor diet. You could find yourself struggling to keep up with the workload, have trouble meeting deadlines, and you could have a hard time socially, too.

It takes courage to live with shyness!
Practical experience of a better diet soon frees you from any suspicion that shyness is weakness. Your 'comfort zone' can extend remarkably quickly, and again, it happens automatically as your diet improves.

We need more education in nutrition

A simple, practical understanding of nutrition, of how to make food work for you, can give you more control over your life than you could ever imagine. Plato, the ancient philosopher, practised good nutrition, he taught it to his students, and his work has stood the test of time. Dr Hay remarked that if the average school or university understood the effect of good nutrition on students, it would have a prominent place on every course.

BEAT PANIC ATTACKS

Change your diet—change your life!

Modern medicine does not always have the complete solution to unexplained anxiety and panic attacks because, as we have seen, it does not work holistically, on mind and body together. Knowing little about nutrition, health professionals can often only treat the symptoms. They can help you to handle the fear, but it cannot disappear altogether until you treat the underlying causes, some of which may well lie in your diet. Hard work, patience and determination are the way to a new life.

DO YOU SUFFER FROM . . .

social phobia?
agoraphobia?
panic in certain other situations?
The possibilities are endless and different for everyone.

Severe anxiety is commoner than anyone realises because we somehow manage to hide it. Persistent panic attacks are not usually under conscious control and have no apparent connection to food, but again they may be largely due to low blood sugar levels, blood sugar swings and hypo attacks. As you work on your diet the overall level of anxiety diminishes and the panic attacks become less intense. Have patience, it can sometimes take a long time.

MORE HELP IN STRESSFUL CIRCUMSTANCES

You will find other natural remedies very much more effective once any problems in your diet have been sorted out.

Stress relief—from a magnet!

A special magnet worn on the wrist like a watch can sometimes relieve background anxiety and stress to a remarkable degree, and the effect can be almost instantaneous. It took me a long time to convince myself that such a simple thing could possibly be helping me so much. But magnets have actually been used in medicine for hundreds of years.

Paracelsus believed in the therapeutic power of magnetism

181

and Father Hall, an eighteenth-century Viennese physician, actually used magnets to treat nervous disorders. A magnet will often also relieve arthritis and all kinds of other problems, even in animals! Most suppliers offer a trial period with a money-back guarantee. See Useful Addresses for supplier.

WARNING: A magnet can ruin a wristwatch, so wear it on the other arm. A magnet will also spoil computer disks.

Flower power

Bach Flower Remedies are homoeopathic remedies which can work powerfully on emotional states: they were especially developed for this purpose. You just find the remedy which suits your personality and symptom picture best. They do not work for everyone, but they are harmless and inexpensive and when they do work they can be astonishingly potent. They can help anyone, children especially, even if they are unwilling to change their diet. They can also combat the effects of food intolerance and have been known to relieve shyness and inhibitions to a considerable extent.

Inner Harmony through Bach Flowers by Sigrid Schmidt is a simple, inexpensive and beautifully illustrated guide. It will enable you to select the correct remedy for you as an individual.

BEAT DEPRESSION

Depression and anxiety go together

You can often find relief from everyday depression by working on your diet. The Hay diet and blood sugar control will gradually raise your spirits, and greatly improve the prospect of getting back to the person you used to be and to the life you once had. Changing my diet gave me a new and much more kindly perspective on life. You have to experience it to believe it.

DO YOU SUFFER FROM DEPRESSION?

Do you feel ...
lost and alone?
that no one cares?
unreasonably guilty about things?
unattractive and worthless?
that you can't cope at times?

Depression is the height of loneliness
Is life cold, bleak and empty?
Is it hard to be alone with your thoughts?
Are you better in company?

A negative attitude is part of the illness!
You think the worst of people.
At times you hate yourself and everyone else.
You see everything and everybody in a bad light.
At times you feel mean and spiteful.
Despite your best intentions, your 'lower self' gets the
better of you.

**These are often only symptoms
They can be reversed!**

When do I get results?

The Hay diet usually begins to calm and revive most people
within just one or two weeks. But changes brought about by
diet can be subtle, and at first you may feel that nothing much
is happening. In fact, other people may see the change in you
before you do. Looking back some time later, you could find to
your surprise that several different problems have definitely
gone. So unless you write the symptoms down before you start
you may well forget you ever had some of them, and abandon
the diet. Keeping a record encourages you to carry on.

But don't expect nature to work to order!
Nervous symptoms are often the last to disappear. So if you are changing your diet to steady your nerves, write down all your physical symptoms, too, and cross them off as they disappear. You may find, for example, that headaches or period pains are first to go, so be patient, the body has its own agenda.

Are you ready to change your life?
Nutritional medicine, beginning with the Hay diet, can work powerfully on the mind. It can work fast and it can work whatever the problem—whether you suffer from unexplained social phobia, agoraphobia, chronic anxiety and depression, or a mixture of the whole lot and more. That seems an extravagant claim to make, and it can be a step in the dark at first, but the results very soon justify your faith in it.

Are you allergic?
DO YOU SUFFER FROM FOOD INTOLERANCE?

Did you know that several of today's antidepressant drugs were originally developed to control the symptoms of allergy?

Removing foods to which you are intolerant further assists the body to heal the mind. See chapter 9.

Are you taking antidepressants or tranquillisers long term?

If you have been taking powerful drugs of any kind long term, the road to recovery could be considerably longer and harder, and your recovery could be less complete, but you can still improve the quality of your life tremendously. Remember that it is essential to wait until you have recovered much of your strength before you consider reducing any drugs, then cut them down very slowly indeed under medical supervision.

BE CAREFUL! Remember that cutting drugs down too quickly can be devastating and could set you back a long way.

MEGA STRESS

I've never been the same since . . .

. . . my baby was born . . . I lost my husband . . . I lost my job . . . I got divorced . . .

A severe shock to the system can so deplete vital reserves of nutrients that the Hay diet and a strong multivitamin and mineral supplement programme are essential. We need supernutrition if we are to survive the shock and exhaustion in the best possible shape and minimise repercussions later.

Chocolate is the last thing we need at times like this!
Remember that stress itself lowers blood sugar and creates a

COMFORT FOODS ADD INSULT TO INJURY
If we overindulge in sweet foods and stimulants
**The body never gets the message
that the emergency is over**
AND THE PANIC AND TIREDNESS CONTINUE

---

craving for sugar and stimulants. So keep your blood sugar level steady with regular meals and frequent snacks of natural food. By eating carelessly at times like this we leave our body to struggle alone. Natural healing is greatly accelerated when the mind consciously co-operates with the body in its efforts to heal.

All your defences down

Shock drastically increases the risk of infection. Any infection could hit you very hard indeed, and without nutritional help your recovery from it could be slow, so again keep your immunity boosted with the Hay diet and supplement programme from the beginning. This is a vital preventative measure and you will be astonished by its power.

THE OTHER NATURAL THERAPIES CAN HELP, TOO

You may well recover faster with the additional help of a homoeopath or a herbalist. Many people also find acupuncture or reflexology surprisingly energising, and they can work almost immediately.

BEAT CHRONIC POST-NATAL DEPRESSION

Childbirth can be mentally and physically devastating, especially if you were unfit, depressed or unwell before the pregnancy started. A foetus takes its nourishment at the mother's expense if necessary, so it can leave you drained for a long time afterwards. Post-natal depression can sometimes become chronic and drag on for months or years without nutritional help.

Take good care of yourself

Life with a young baby is hectic, and a mother may neglect her diet at a time when she really needs supernutrition to build herself up and keep the baby well supplied with breast milk. You can achieve tremendous relief in a surprisingly short time on the Hay diet, blood sugar control and extra vitamins and minerals.

Long-standing post-natal depression

If the symptoms do not improve substantially, look for the underlying cause. Consider allergy, candida and mercury toxicity.

Could your baby be allergic?
Mothers with chronic post-natal illness who find they have nutritional problems such as food intolerance, often find that the baby inherits them. So if a baby is fretful and hard to manage, read the information on allergic children in chapter 10.

Preventing post-natal illness

If at all possible, sort out your diet and get fit *before* you become pregnant. Foresight is an organisation which takes a nutritional approach and which publishes several very helpful books. Their address is at the end of the book.

ANITA'S STORY
I've been SO tired since my baby was born. I've been eating lots of sugar to keep my energy up, but I get so tired in the evenings that I can't even concentrate on TV. The doctor said it could take three years to get back to normal; he said there was nothing he could do. Well, I've cut out the tea and all the sugar and sweet things and I feel SO much better already. I've only been on the Hay diet a few days and I feel SO good!

DEBBIE'S STORY
Debbie had two babies. She woke up tired and tearful and pushed herself through the day. She had trembling attacks and severe anxiety, aggressive outbursts, sleeping problems, nightmares, sore throats and hot and cold sweats. She was drinking lots of tea with three spoonfuls of sugar in every cup, and she snacked all day—on chocolate, biscuits, white bread, fruit and chips. She fed the children very well, but she never had a proper meal at all herself, except on Sundays.

With her mother's dedicated help, after just nine days on the Hay diet and blood sugar control, Debbie's husband rang to say, 'She's right down to one cup of tea a day, she eats salads, wholemeal bread and natural food, and the panics have all

187

gone. She's great, she's brilliant!. And I feel much better myself on this diet, so you've done me a favour, too.'

──────── *HOLISTIC ANXIETY MANAGEMENT* ────────

A Master Plan

1   The Hay diet.
2   Learn to control your blood sugar levels.
3   Follow the vitamin and mineral supplement programme.
4   Identify any food intolerances.
5   Consider candida if you still feel unwell.
6   Make sure you take enough rest.
7   Reduce your stressload/workload if you can.
8   If recovery is slow, consider mercury toxicity.

CHAPTER 13

Get Your Fats Right

Not all fat is bad for us by any means. Fats make up around 30 per cent of our body weight and the right fats are essential to almost every bodily function. Everyone needs a plentiful supply of certain fats and oils, and good health really depends on knowing which fats are good and which are bad. Some fats are made in the body, but there are others which the body cannot make, and they must be taken in food every single day. These are known as the 'essential fats'. They are essential to everyone, slimmers included, and they are abundant in fresh, natural food.

Low-fat diets which lack essential fats and oils are a serious health hazard

We are right to limit the saturated animal fats from dairy products and meat, but many of us are also restricting the essential fats and oils and this is making us ill, with a wide range of problems, both physical and mental. If we do not take enough essential oils, the body does the best it can with the fat it is given, however unsuitable. Animal fats have long been known to clog the arteries if we take too much, but transfats are an even bigger menace, and hardly anyone is aware of the danger. These are polyunsaturated vegetable fats which have been damaged by heavy processing to prolong their shelf life in the shops. They then behave like saturated fats, but they put us at even greater risk because, unlike animal fats, they are unknown in nature and completely unnatural to the body.

TRANSFATS ARE DEAD, DISTORTED AND DANGEROUS

They do more harm than the saturated fat they are intended to replace.

They are found in:

- Deep-fried snacks.
- Bakery goods and confectionery.
- Ordinary supermarket cooking oils.
- Margarines (hydrogenated fat is transfat).

Transfats are toxic and contribute to:

- Greasy skin, spots, pimples, acne, blackheads.
- Greasy hair that needs washing often.
- Overweight, cellulite.
- Heart problems, high blood pressure.
- Cancer.

But when transfats are replaced with natural food containing essential fats, the body soon gets to work repairing the damage.

ESSENTIAL OILS FOR SOFTNESS AND FLEXIBILITY

The richest sources of essential oils are:

- Natural unrefined oils of all kinds.
- Fresh oily fish, fruit, nuts and seeds.
- Avocado pears, fresh vegetables and salads.

**A BODY THAT LACKS ESSENTIAL OILS
WILL BE DRY!**

- A dry mouth, thirst.
- Dry lips that are sore in winter.
- A dry skin that ages more quickly.
- Stiff, dry, clicky and creaky joints.
- Painful tendons that have lost their elasticity.
- Dry eyes.

**TRANSFATS ADD TO THE GENERAL DRYNESS
OF THE BODY**
They prevent essential fats from being absorbed

The absorption of essential fats is blocked by:

- Too much saturated fat.
- Refined sugar.
- Alcohol.
- Stress.

Essential fats help to make up the sheaths of all our nerves
Lack of them can therefore cause nerve pains and neurological problems of all kinds. Thirty per cent of the brain also consists of essential fats, so a deficiency can lead to any number of nervous and mental problems.

ESSENTIAL OILS ARE BIOLOGICALLY ACTIVE

Here are some more of the jobs they do around the body:

- They condition the skin and hair without making them greasy.
- They condition the mucous membranes throughout the body.

WHAT WILL ESSENTIAL OILS DO FOR ME?

Glossy hair and clearer, softer skin
Increased vitality
Sounder sleep
Improved joint mobility
Improved mental functioning

In the longer term

Greater resistance to sunburn
Tougher, thicker skin—not so easily broken
Increased muscle and tendon elasticity, relief from
tendon pain
Substantial improvement in arthritis
Dry, clicking and creaking joints are lubricated
They help to prevent osteoporosis

YOU CAN ALSO OBTAIN SURPRISING RELIEF FROM:

Anxiety, tension
Insomnia
Hormone problems, PMT, breast pain
Nerve pains anywhere, even in the teeth
Acne, eczema
Allergies and food intolerance
Nervous problems of all kinds
Dry pimply skin, dry eyes
A sore, irritable bladder
Skin problems of all kinds
Low blood sugar

- They make flexible, healthy cell membranes which can screen out impurities.
- They allow the passage of waste material from cells.
- They are essential to the formation of bile salts in the liver. Bile salts help to digest fatty food.
- They are part of the structure of our hormones, including the sex hormones, especially testosterone.
- Enzymes break down food ready for absorption, and a quarter of all our enzyme systems depend on fats.
- They keep the red blood cells soft and flexible, so that they do not stick together and form clots.
- They control the levels of triglycerides and cholesterol. Vegetable fats are cholesterol free.
- The absorption of fat-soluble nutrients from the intestine depends on essential oils.

It is also likely that levels of essential fats in early life help to determine future health.

* * *

Remember that we need plenty of salad to ensure we get the high intake of vitamins and minerals which enable the body to utilise the oil.

Ordinary refined cooking oil

The refining of natural oils is a disaster for all of us, comparable with the refining of sugar and wholemeal flour. Besides containing transfats, the natural antioxidant, which is vitamin E, is processed out of natural oil and replaced by chemical antioxidants to prevent rancidity. The vitamin E is then sold in capsules in health food shops.

TAKE YOUR SALAD WITH OIL, IT'S ESSENTIAL

Extra virgin olive oil
Light sesame oil
Sunflower oil, safflower oil
Corn oil, walnut oil

Vary the oils
Each oil adds its own special flavour
One or two teaspoonfuls of oil per serving is enough

* * *

**ORDINARY REFINED
SUPERMARKET VEGETABLE OILS ARE
NOT SUITABLE FOR SALADS**
because they contain transfats
Use only natural unrefined or cold pressed oils
from a health food shop

OLIVE OIL

All the natural unrefined oils contain polyunsaturated, monounsaturated and saturated fats in varying proportions. Extra virgin olive oil is highest in monounsaturated fat. The medicinal properties of extra virgin olive oil have been celebrated since ancient times, but the way it works is still something of a mystery. Mediterranean people who use it certainly suffer less heart disease than we do, and it has worked wonders for my skin, relieved my tendon pain and helped me put on weight.

FLAX SEED OR LINSEED OIL (OMEGA 3 OIL)

Flax is being cultivated commercially on a large scale now. You may have seen it growing, the fields a mass of dainty blue flowers. The seeds are pressed to make linseed oil.

ARE YOU DEFICIENT IN OMEGA 3 OILS?

Depression	Dry skin
Heart problems	Fluid retention
High blood cholesterol	High blood pressure
Inflammation anywhere	Poor vision
Poor co-ordination	Slow growth in children
Poor immunity	Poor memory, poor learning ability

Omega 3 oil is often lacking in cases of schizophrenia

Linseed oil can be used instead of fish oil

Food grade linseed oil is available in capsules and in bottles. The bottled oil works out cheaper than the capsules and is more effective. If you are very deficient in essential fats you may need 1–3 teaspoonfuls daily. For a supplier, see Useful Addresses.

Where else do I find Omega 3 oils?
Fresh nuts, sunflower, sesame and pumpkin seeds.

Fish oil is also Omega 3

It is found in fresh oily fish such as sardines, mackerel and herrings. We need two helpings of oily fish per week or any ONE of these instead:

- 1 teaspoonful cod liver oil per day, *or*
- 1 teaspoonful linseed oil per day. *or*
- 1–3 × 1g EPA fish oil concentrate capsules per day. This oil is from the body of an oily fish, not the liver.

─── *WE NEED BOTH OMEGA 3 AND OMEGA 6 OILS* ───

EVENING PRIMROSE OIL OR GLA (GAMMA LINOLEIC ACID—OMEGA 6 OIL)

The power of high doses of evening primrose oil is well known. It is also an extremely effective natural tranquilliser and a marvellous tonic with a huge range of other benefits.

How does it work?

It replenishes the brain with essential fatty acids, and can therefore help any mental or nervous problem. Essential fats form part of every cell in the body, which explains their wide-ranging benefits.

- It may be several weeks before you feel the benefit of it, because it can take time to build up in the system, depending on how deficient you are.
- If you cannot take it by mouth, snip the end off the capsule and rub the oil onto any soft area of skin (not directly onto any area of eczema).
- Take 1–3g per day. If you are very deficient you could start with a high dose and reduce it as the symptoms improve.
- If you suffer from temporal lobe epilepsy or schizophrenia consult your doctor before taking evening primrose oil.

VITAMIN E—NATURAL D ALPHA TOCOPHEROL (OIL CAPSULES)

If you are taking extra oil, natural vitamin E 100 units will help to prevent it turning rancid in the body. For faster and better results, keep to the Hay diet.

THINGS PEOPLE SAY
I've had a 'heavy head' for years, and two tablespoonfuls of olive oil each morning have solved the problem.

After a short time on 3g evening primrose oil a day, I could see better, hear better and sleep sounder. It's magic.

I used to have to wash and style my hair every single day. But now I'm on the Hay diet it doesn't get greasy, and it's so much easier to manage.

I've had these awful migraines for years, and now at last I've found the cause—it was evening primrose oil, I am allergic to it!

MAKE THE FAT CONNECTION
The Hay diet enhances and accelerates the effect of all the oils
Always include extra virgin olive oil in the diet, 1–2 tablespoons daily

---

SAFETY NOTE: Evening primrose oil, linseed oil, fish oil and vitamin E all tend to thin the blood, so be careful not to take them to excess if you are taking blood-thinning medication such as aspirin or Warfarin. There is more very helpful information in *A Consumer Guide to Vitamins* by Angela Dowden and Grahame Lacey.

DRY SKIN
Most skin problems will respond to the Hay diet plus extra oils. You can soften and waterproof the skin quite considerably in a short time. Olive oil can be rubbed into the skin if you dislike the taste.

THIN SKIN
When transfats are built into the skin, it becomes drier, coarser and thinner, and it grazes easily if you fall over. The Hay diet and essential fats can work wonders for your skin over the

years. The skin on my hands doesn't usually graze any more, and now I can be touched. If your skin is thin you instinctively react to touch by drawing away.

BREAST PAIN
Where there is a lack of essential fats, fibrous tissue and cysts are more likely to form. The Hay diet with the right kind of fats helps to avoid worrying lumps in the breast and can sometimes alleviate the pain and reduce the inflammation and tenderness. Higher rates of breast cancer have been noted in countries where the intake of dairy fats is high.

HORMONE PROBLEMS AND PMT
It is well known that evening primrose oil can be a great help in PMT. The Hay diet enhances and accelerates its effect.

OSTEOPOROSIS
Essential oils help to absorb calcium from the gut.

HARDENING OF THE ARTERIES
Essential oils build living, breathing cells with soft and flexible walls. Too much transfat and too little essential oils means that many of the cells built into artery walls will be hard and rigid, but with the right kind of fats the body begins to repair the damage.

ASTHMA AND ECZEMA
When transfats are built into the walls of the breathing tubes they get wheezy and prone to infection because the mucous membranes get so out of condition. A lack of essential oils is common to both asthma and eczema. They can respond extremely well to the Hay diet and essential oils.

ALZHEIMER'S DISEASE

Lack of essential fats can be a contributory factor. Memory has been known to improve when they are supplied.

IRRITABLE BOWEL, CANDIDA, COLITIS

When the mucous membrane of the bowel is in poor condition it leaves us open to irritation and infection.

SORE, IRRITABLE BLADDER

Again, unhealthy mucous membrane becomes prone to irritation and infection.

STIFF JOINTS? GET SUPPLE AGAIN!

If you lie down on your back, knees bent, feet together, and see how far you can comfortably open your legs, you will probably find it will not be very far, especially if you are middle-aged or older, but plenty of natural oils will help to keep you moving. Body tissues become softer and more elastic. The whole body becomes more supple and flexible.

CANCER

Unlike healthy cells which screen toxins out, when transfats are built into cell walls they admit toxins, increasing the risk of cancer.

LOW RESISTANCE TO INFECTION

The immune system needs essential oils because the white blood cells that fight infection must be soft and flexible if they are to engulf and digest harmful bacteria.

On a restricted diet for candida or food intolerance?
You may find that you are by now extremely deficient in essential fats. *Evening Primrose Oil* by Judy Graham is comprehensive and very helpful in explaining how it works and how much to take in these and many other conditions.

LOW BODY TEMPERATURE

Many of us are unnaturally cold and would love to be more comfortable. Here are some suggestions which may help:

- Eat regularly, snack often.
- Keep your blood sugar level steady.
- Make sure you get enough to eat during the day.
- Make sure you get plenty of natural vegetable oils. Fats and carbohydrates eaten together produce warmth.
- Remember that repeated or prolonged low calorie diets and missing meals slow metabolism.
- Mercury can sometimes lower body temperature.
- Thyroid problems can lower body temperature too. The GP can test your blood for thyroid deficiency.

Replenish your carbohydrate reserves every morning

Blood sugar levels drop overnight and I have learnt to combat morning chill by repeated starchy snacks like porridge, blended with olive oil, alternating with fresh fruit or salad, until I feel warm again.

CHAPTER 14

Vitamin Power

Knowing little about vitamins, and having no experience of taking them in high doses, we tend to assume that compared with drugs they must surely be weak and ineffectual. Nothing could be farther from the truth. Most people are very surprised indeed at their power, and history confirms it. Children in misery from the pain of rickets, cured by the vitamin D in cod liver oil; sailors dying of scurvy, cured by the vitamin C in lemon juice—that is vitamin power! But doctors had no scientific understanding of how these foods worked until many years later, when vitamins were discovered.

NOTHING CHANGES
Vitamins and minerals are still the raw material of healing. They are the substances the body is most familiar with, and knows exactly how to use. And in suitable doses their effects are wide-ranging and can be astonishingly beneficial.

DRUGS OBSTRUCT NATURAL HEALING
Antibiotics overcome infections artificially. By contrast, high-dose vitamins and minerals, together with essential oils, give the body the extra resources to deal with infection by itself, in its own way, and for everyday infections they can work surprisingly well.

Only nature can cure

Drugs are chemicals; they cannot rebuild body cells, but nature can. Chronic illness usually responds far more quickly to natural medicine, beginning with the Hay diet, because food is the only material the body can use to repair itself. The vitamins, minerals, and all the other nutrients present in food gradually fortify the whole system until it can function without support. But many of us have become so deficient over the years that we cannot get enough nutrients from food alone, so vitamin and mineral supplements are required to speed recovery.

THIS IS A POWERFUL SUPPLEMENT PROGRAMME

Take once a day at mealtimes
One extra-strong multivitamin and mineral tablet containing at least 25mg vitamin B complex

Twice a day
Vitamin C one gram (1,000 mg)

Two or three times a day
Evening primrose oil 1G
(1g = 2 × 500mg capsules)

Gradually reduce the supplements when you feel better

This programme will rapidly boost your vitality, it is mentally calming and a very powerful tonic. As you become accustomed to using it, together with the Hay diet, your confidence in natural medicine will grow by leaps and bounds. If you are sceptical and reluctant to change your diet, you could perhaps try making the vitamin connection first. The results of this programme will certainly make you think!

A powerful way of dealing with stress
Stress rapidly drains us of vitamins and minerals, so you might like to keep some supplements ready for emergency use:

- To combat shock or an emotional upset.
- Before an interview, a day out, anything which drains you physically or mentally.

Protect yourself from infection

- If you feel an infection coming on you can nip it in the bud.
- If someone at home has an infection, you can take them to prevent you catching it.
- They speed recovery from absolutely any illness.

Make sure you take a high enough dose.

Ordinary vitamin and mineral tablets, those containing just the RDA (recommended daily allowance), are not nearly strong enough for people who are unwell.

- Quest SUPER Once a Day multivitamin and mineral tablets contain 50mg vitamin B complex plus 10mg zinc and are very widely available.
- It is safer and less expensive to take multivitamin and mineral tablets which also contain all eleven B vitamins, because vitamins and minerals work best together as a team, and vitamins depend on minerals for their absorption.

Sublingual vitamins are taken under the tongue, where absorption is extremely high. People with gut and malabsorption problems can find them tremendously helpful.
If vitamin tablets cause you problems, food state vitamins may be easier to tolerate. They are better absorbed, so you can benefit from a lower dose.

Buy your vitamins from a health food shop

If you buy them from a health food shop they will not contain unnecessary colours or additives. They are manufactured by food supplement companies and some may actually be available on medical prescription in Britain. Ask your pharmacist as the situation is changing all the time.

SOME IMPORTANT POINTS

Vitamin A is stored and can build up to an overdose in the body

Apart from the dose in multivitamin tablets, it is also abundant as beta-carotene in fruit and vegetables, especially those that are dark green, red, yellow and orange. The body turns beta-carotene to vitamin A. Cod liver oil is rich in vitamins A and D.

Too much vitamin A can cause:

- Dry skin and hair, sore eyes, irritability, headaches and joint pain.
- And did you know that a four-ounce slice of lamb's liver may contain up to 28,000 units of vitamin A!

So make sure you take plenty of extra virgin olive oil with salad—to ensure its proper absorption.

Vitamin D is also stored in the body, but overdose is unlikely

It is found in liver, oily fish, eggs and dairy products but not in fruit and vegetables. The body also manufactures its own vitamin D under the skin when exposed to sunlight.

CAUTION: Large or long-continued doses of one individual vitamin or mineral can sometimes throw the rest out of balance, which can be dangerous.

ARE YOU DEFICIENT IN ZINC?

Zinc deficiency is incredibly common. Most debilitated people are deficient in zinc. It is depleted from the soil by artificial fertilisers, and is processed out of many foods, especially sugar, white flour and white rice. Mercury, too, robs us of zinc.

ZINC DEFICIENCY PLAYS A PART IN:

Depression	Allergies
Poor mental function	Hormone problems
Poor appetite	Poor sense of taste and smell
Food cravings	Skin problems
Eating disorders	Slow healing of wounds
Low resistance to infection	Mental and physical tiredness

IMPROVEMENT CAN BE RAPID AND VERY SURPRISING

It can sometimes take several weeks to replenish yourself.
Take 5–15mg zinc citrate per day
and taste-test at least once a week.

**Are you taking the stronger multivitamin
and mineral tablets?**
If they contain up to 15mg of zinc do not take any more.

ZINCATEST is a zinc solution, a taste-test for zinc deficiency, available from health food shops or directly from Lamberts food supplement company. If you are deficient you cannot taste anything at all. When you are able to taste the zinc you will have had enough. *The Zinc Solution* by Dr Derek Bryce Smith contains more valuable information.

You will get to know when your zinc level is dropping, because the symptoms come back. You may, for example, crave food or be less able to taste it. Many people find they have to continue taking zinc indefinitely, every day, otherwise their symptoms return.

You can take too much zinc

We can only absorb a certain amount every day—individuals vary. I get dizzy if I take too much. Sometimes people react to zinc initially, with palpitations, for example, but as they recover their health they are able to take a little and increase it gradually, as I did myself.

ARE YOU ANAEMIC?

If you are always pale and often tired, a little extra iron could work wonders. It increases the oxygen in the blood and can produce many improvements throughout the body. Iron deficiency can also contribute to poor concentration, headaches, irritability and dizziness. Haemoglobin checks for iron deficiency are available from GP surgeries.

Spatone Iron + is iron-rich spa water from a Welsh spring
It is gentle, non-constipating and very easily absorbed. It comes in sachets: I empty the contents into a small bottle and take a teaspoonful each day. It has put colour in my cheeks for the first time ever. See Useful Addresses for supplier.

You can take too much iron

The ordinary iron supplements from the pharmacy are a much stronger dose.

A DEFICIENCY OF VITAMIN B COMPLEX

The B vitamins are abundant in natural foods, especially fresh vegetables, but they are very easily destroyed by cooking. This is our most common vitamin deficiency because B vitamins are also stripped from sugar, white rice and white bread in the refining process. It is a big problem nowadays, even amongst children, because our diets are so full of highly processed foods and sweet drinks, and because we eat so little fresh fruit and salad. Mental symptoms appear first because the B vitamins are so essential to brain function, and when supplements are taken, the improvement in mental function can sometimes be quite remarkable.

- The B vitamins also combat anxiety and depression and release energy from carbohydrate foods.

ARE YOU DEFICIENT IN VITAMIN B COMPLEX?

These are some of the symptoms:

Depression	Anxiety
Mental tiredness	Fatigue, low energy
Poor concentration	Muscle weakness
Short attention-span	Poor appetite
Poor short-term memory	Indigestion
Grumpy and antisocial	Skin problems
Cracked and fissured tongue	Allergies
Falling hair	Chronic fatigue

SYMPTOMS LIKE THIS ARE TOO
EASILY ACCEPTED
Vitamin B complex is best taken as part of a
multivitamin and mineral supplement as suggested in
the supplement programme on p. 202

What contributes to B deficiency?

Sugar and sweet foods	White flour
Alcohol	White rice
Stress	Contraceptive pills
Candida	Psychiatric drugs
Antibiotics	Hormone replacement therapy

Make sure you take the whole of the B complex
There are eleven different vitamins in the whole B complex, and they are all found in the vitamin and mineral tablets recommended on p. 203. You may find that it turns your urine bright yellow but this is harmless: it is due to excess vitamins being excreted in the urine.

DRUG DEPENDENCE CAN OFTEN BE REDUCED

Many people's health continues to deteriorate over the years despite drug treatment, and the symptoms come back if they stop the drugs. Nutritional therapy, beginning with the Hay diet, can halt and then gradually reverse the disease process, steadily restoring lost function to the body as a whole. You may gradually be able to reduce any drugs as you recover your strength.

Drugs can be lifesavers in a crisis, but by suppressing symptoms artificially rather than assisting the body to deal with its own problems in its own way, as diet and supplements do, they obstruct natural healing in the long term. Consequently we become progressively weaker, and less able to overcome illness naturally. People taking drugs long term usually experience a downward spiral of ill health as I did myself. But the Hay diet and nutritional therapy provide a huge range of benefits, without penalties.

My own experience of being ill, my long journey back to health, and all my research since, have convinced me that the safest and quickest way to recover from chronic health problems, whether they are mental or physical, is by natural methods, beginning with the Hay diet. Any attempt to fix things artificially with drugs alone leads to more trouble in the long term.

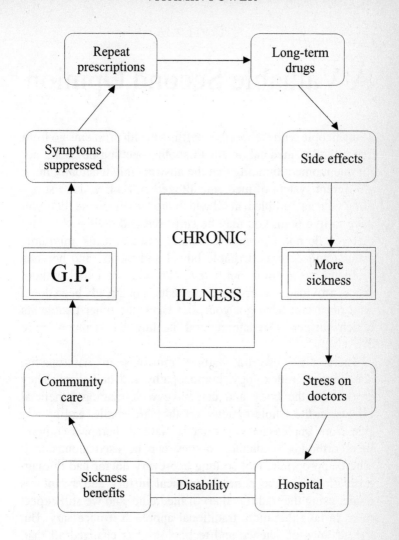

CHAPTER 15

A Valuable Second Opinion

Many people with stubborn or baffling health problems go from one orthodox medical doctor to another, getting nowhere, not for one moment thinking that the answers might actually lie in a different system of medicine altogether. So if you are struggling with any problem at all which modern medicine feels you have to live with, you may be surprised and delighted to find that you do not. Common complaints like arthritis, migraine, asthma and eczema, irritable bowel and mental and nervous problems, to mention but a few, can often be cured without drugs, provided irreversible damage has not already been done. And once you have got your diet right, the other treatments which further stimulate natural healing work much more effectively.

There are powerful natural remedies in naturopathy, acupuncture, reflexology, homoeopathy and herbalism. They work with the body and can have wide-ranging beneficial effects on the whole system, yet they are gentle, and largely free from unpleasant side-effects. Natural therapies complement orthodox medicine, so they can be used alongside it where appropriate. Not so long ago every doctor had to diagnose illness on the patient's medical history and symptoms alone, using the traditional art of medicine, and we still expect them to take this more traditional approach if necessary. But the advance of science and technology has changed all that: medicine today is largely scientific, and treatment is based on laboratory tests and the availability of suitable drugs; it is restricted to what can be scientifically understood.

So whatever happened to the art of medicine?
It is alive and well. The natural health practitioners are using it today just as doctors did before the development of science and technology. A visit to a natural health practitioner can be surprisingly helpful. The first consultation usually lasts at least an hour, and you will find that he or she asks the right questions, listens, and believes you. These practitioners are mainly the arts people, sensitive, intuitive and practical. The anecdotal evidence which doctors so often dismiss is vital to them, it makes good sense. They rely on your experience for the diagnosis and the response to treatment. Naturopathy and nutritional therapy, in particular, are a common-sense blend of art and science.

NATUROPATHS
Otherwise known as naturopathic physicians, naturopaths can examine their own patients, make diagnoses and can issue sickness certificates recognised in Britain by the Departments of Health and Social Security. They concentrate on improving general health without the use of drugs, mainly by detoxifying the body. They look at the whole picture—diet, lifestyle, stress, everything. They use herbal remedies, hydrotherapy and exercise. Many are also qualified osteopaths or acupuncturists. In North America naturopaths work under the supervision of a medical practitioner.

NUTRITIONAL THERAPY
Diets and vitamin and mineral supplements are used to treat most everyday complaints and can have remarkable success, especially with chronic conditions, both physical and mental.

ACUPUNCTURE
This is a safe treatment which can have a rapid and powerful tonic effect on the whole system, and raise energy levels very considerably. Very fine needles are used to relieve pain and to stimulate healing. And where traditional acupuncture fails,

electro-acupuncture may well succeed, as it did for me. A mild electric current is passed through the needles. Acupuncture is becoming more widely available on the health services, in GP surgeries and especially in hospital pain clinics.

REFLEXOLOGY AND FOOD INTOLERANCE

Reflexology treats pressure points on the feet which correspond to specific parts of the body. Like acupuncture, it can considerably raise energy levels. *My many food intolerances have improved remarkably since having reflexology twice weekly, now continuing once a week.*

HOMOEOPATHY

It has been known for centuries that minute doses of medicine can stimulate the immune system and activate the healing response in a powerful way. It is worth a try because some people respond amazingly well. Homoeopathy is available on the British National Health Service on a limited basis. Many general practitioners are also homoeopaths.

SCEPTICAL?

We dislike simple answers; we distrust them and frequently dismiss them without further thought. Scientific minds in particular often find it hard to take a holistic view of illness, being naturally more concerned with detail and scientific proof. Such differing attitudes to solving health problems spring from fundamental and opposing differences in human nature. But we need the best of both worlds if we are to be well. Natural medicine is diametrically opposed to orthodox medicine in many ways; it is based on a different set of beliefs. It is non-specific: treatment is not aimed at any particular symptom but supports the body generally, giving it the strength to sort out its own problems in its own way. It works on observation and experience, it is based on practical acquaintance with the facts. Modern medicine deals with the effects of illness, it treats the symptoms, but natural medicine sees symptoms in a quite different light. It treats them as alarm calls, intelligent signals from a body in distress, and supports the body in its efforts to heal itself. By suppressing the symptoms, drugs switch off the alarm without putting out the fire. And in the long term this leads to chronic illness, disability and endless expense.

Partners in care

Complementary medicine recognises that disease develops over a long time, and by dealing with the early warning symptoms, it seeks to halt and reverse it. Modern medicine deals with the symptoms of illness when it has already developed, when the damage has been done. It deals best with the crises. The two systems of medicine complement each other perfectly.

If simple remedies were tried before drugs, complementary methods would lead the field in everyday medicine. The fact that they are safe and are found to work is proof enough for most of us. If everyone were taught the full facts about nutrition, as the World Health Organisation recommends, far fewer drugs would be needed. As things stand, we know next to nothing about food in relation to the way we feel, and today's diet is a recipe for disaster.

MEDICINE HAS CHANGED

Medical research into the causes of illness had a good track record before drugs became so freely available. It found answers to scurvy, rickets, beri-beri and pellagra. They all proved to be just vitamin deficiencies, and when they were corrected the results were spectacular. Doctors in those days knew where to look for the answers. Such research still goes on, and many more such treatments have been discovered.

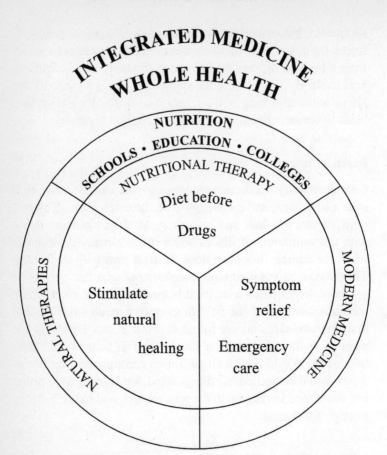

INTEGRATED MEDICINE
WHOLE HEALTH

NUTRITION

SCHOOLS · EDUCATION · COLLEGES

NUTRITIONAL THERAPY

Diet before

Drugs

NATURAL THERAPIES

MODERN MEDICINE

Stimulate

natural

healing

Symptom

relief

Emergency

care

Truth never dies

These methods are still being used by a tiny band of pioneer doctors, humanitarians such as Dr Abraham Hoffer in Canada. Over the last 40 years he has been quietly curing mental illness, including many of his schizophrenic patients. He sees schizo-phrenia as a form of pellagra, a deficiency of niacin, which is vitamin B3. But despite its success, his work is largely ignored. How differently these discoveries would have been received in days gone by. This is the kind of medicine we understand,

214

these are the methods we trust. By trying to impose its beliefs on the natural order, orthodox medicine is losing its way.

A REVOLUTION IN THE TREATMENT OF MENTAL ILLNESS

It has now also been discovered that many other people have extraordinarily high requirements for certain vitamins and minerals, and that specific supplements can restore the balance of their minds. This is ortho-molecular medicine, and there has been astonishing success with mental problems of all kinds, from depression and anxiety to manic depression, just by investigating the diet and individual body chemistry and making the necessary adjustments. Doctors who specialise in allergy and nutritional medicine may be able to help. See Useful Addresses. There is also much valuable information in *Mental Health and Mental Illness* by Dr Carl Pfeiffer and Patrick Holford.

CHAPTER 16

Is Mercury Your Problem?

Many people with a long list of mental and physical symptoms have tried everything orthodox and complementary medicine have to offer but still they remain unwell. Many are desperate. Their candida, hypoglycaemia, allergies and many other problems never fully respond to any of the usual treatments and they feel something else must be obstructing their progress. If you have the usual silver or black metal fillings in your teeth it may be worth consulting a dentist who runs a mercury-free dental practice to see if mercury is affecting your general health. There are tests to confirm it.

How does mercury escape from the teeth?

Hot drinks, chewing, brushing your teeth and grinding them during sleep all release mercury vapour. Mercury also infiltrates the tissues surrounding the tooth.

Do you panic over little things?
Do you frequently 'get into a state?' General anxiety, panic, impulsiveness and a tendency to lose your grip at times are typical of mercury sensitivity.

Mercury is highly poisonous

Even at low levels it can have devastating effects. One small filling can sometimes be enough to cause huge problems in very sensitive people, especially children. Pioneering dentist Hal Huggins tells some remarkable stories in *It's All in Your Head*.

EARLY SYMPTOMS OF MERCURY POISONING

Fatigue
Short-term memory loss
Poor concentration
Fears and phobias
Obsessive, compulsive behaviour
Reluctance to tackle mental tasks

Mercury is a neurotoxin, a nerve poison
The roof of the mouth is the floor of the brain
The brain is the first to be affected by mercury
It specifically attacks the short-term memory centre

Mercury amalgam fillings are 50 per cent mercury, which has long been known to be poisonous. Sometimes people can relate the onset of their problems to when they first had their fillings put in, but more often it is a slow, insidious process of mental and physical deterioration which happens over many years. Mercury can accumulate throughout the body, especially in the brain, heart, liver and kidneys. It is excreted in the urine.

WHY IS MERCURY PERMITTED IF IT IS SO TOXIC?

The story begins in the USA, in the 1830s, when the only available filling material was gold. Because it was too expensive for most people, amalgam was developed to satisfy the demand for a cheaper substitute. But the American Society of Dental Surgeons warned people against it and banned the dentists who used it from their membership. So the amalgam users then joined forces to form the American Dental Association, staunch in their defence of mercury amalgam, and they prospered. The British Dental Association is of the same mind: they believe that mercury amalgam is safe for all but a tiny minority of people.

CHRONIC LOW-LEVEL MERCURY POISONING

These are some of the symptoms

Neurological problems	Pins and needles
Unexplained chest pains	Emotional instability
Candida	Poor resistance to infection
Allergies	Bleeding gums
Kidney problems	Low blood sugar
Thyroid problems	Fatigue
Stomach problems	Poor vision
Bowel problems	Raised white blood cell count
Food intolerance	Digestive upsets
Gum problems	Hormone problems
Tinnitus	Headaches
Low sperm count	Shaking
A fast-beating heart	Zinc deficiency
Chemical sensitivities	Memory loss
Infertility	Miscarriages, stillbirths
Hair loss	Abnormal hair growth
Sinus problems	Arthritis
Muscle spasms	Muscle weakness

The World Health Organisation is concerned

In 1991 the WHO published findings that the main source of mercury in the body came from fillings and that the average amalgam filling releases up to half its mercury content over ten years, through corrosion; the most corroded fillings are those which are now black. It also concluded that there is no safe level of mercury vapour. The World Health Organisation is humanitarian and not influenced by business or professional interests.

MORE SYMPTOMS OF MERCURY TOXICITY

Travel sickness	Heart or chest pain
Skin problems of all kinds	Angina
Low blood pressure	High blood pressure
Diarrhoea	Constipation
Shingles	Numbness, tingling anywhere
Poor appetite	Heartburn, bloating
Metallic taste	Swollen glands
Deafness	Increased saliva
Frequent passing of urine	Dizziness
Burning mouth	Excessive sweating
The shakes	Antibiotic resistance
Irregular heartbeat	Mouth ulcers and sores
Pressure round the head	Earache
Blackouts	Low body temperature
Low stomach acid	Numbness
Mental fogging	Poor short-term memory
Slow healing	Body stench
Restricted breathing	Backache

MERCURY VAPOUR SPECIFICALLY TARGETS THE BRAIN

Mercury levels in the brain are in direct proportion to the number of tooth surfaces covered by amalgam fillings. Mercury vapour is being released all the time; it passes straight through the lining of the mouth and nose, crosses the blood-brain barrier designed to protect us from toxins and infection and is transported directly to the brain and spinal cord. 'Mad as a hatter' came into the language when hatters worked with mercury, and dentists have to keep scrap amalgam in special sealed containers to prevent it vaporising!

MERCURY POISONING CAN ALSO BE INVOLVED IN:

Alzheimer's disease	Multiple sclerosis
Depression	Migraine
Suicidal depression	Epilepsy
Leukaemia	Raynaud's syndrome
Lupus erythematosis	Endometriosis
Crohn's disease	Brain cancer
Ulcerative colitis	Chronic fatigue, M.E.
Heart attacks	Hodgkin's disease
Motor neurone disease	Paralysis
Anorexia nervosa	Alcoholism
Parkinson's disease	Bell's palsy
Glandular fever	Schizophrenia
Sickle cell anaemia	Diabetes
Asthma	Severe emotional problems

THIS LIST IS BY NO MEANS COMPLETE!

Mercury is stored in fat

Remember that up to sixty per cent of the brain is made from fats and so are the sheaths of all our nerves, which accounts for the frequent implication of mercury in Alzheimer's disease and multiple sclerosis (MS).

METHYL MERCURY

Bacteria in the mouth interact with mercury to produce methyl mercury, which is one hundred times more neurotoxic than elemental mercury. This is the most dangerous compound of mercury. It contributes to indigestion, stomach pains, peptic ulcers and irritable bowel. It contaminates the saliva and constantly

220

trickles down into the gut, killing the friendly bacteria which control candida. After my own mercury was removed my stomach settled amazingly fast.

Fish contains methyl mercury

If you are unwell and fish affects you badly, this might be part of the reason.

Mercury can affect unborn babies

It crosses the placental barrier, accumulates in the foetus and contaminates breast milk. Mercury levels in the foetus and breast milk are eight times the level present in the mother's body. Having amalgam fillings inserted or removed during pregnancy may release enough mercury vapour to affect the foetus.

NO SMOKE WITHOUT FIRE!

Dentists in California are required to display this warning: 'This office uses amalgam filling materials which contain and expose you to mercury, a chemical known to cause birth defects and other reproductive harm.'

The German government recommends that amalgam should not be used in women of child-bearing age. It also warns against placing mercury amalgam in children under six years old, and people with kidney problems.

In 1998 the British government suggested to doctors and dentists that, as a precautionary measure, mothers should avoid having amalgam fillings removed or replaced during pregnancy.

In Sweden the government will not pay for amalgam fillings. It also pays 70 per cent of the cost of replacing them.

In Austria it is being phased out.

**THERE IS NO POSITIVE PROOF THAT
MERCURY IS SAFE**
There is no research anywhere that positively
demonstrates the safety of dental amalgam as a
non-toxic substance.

MORE ABOUT THE EFFECTS OF MERCURY

Electric currents in the mouth

These are not fully understood. Each tooth is thought to be con-
nected to a specific part of the body via an electrical pathway,
similar to an acupuncture meridian. Electric currents from metals in the mouth can also affect the brain. Negative electric current causes the most mercury to be released.

Electric currents can be measured

An amalgameter is a special probe which registers the current
when it touches the tooth. Mercury-free dentists use one, and
so do some homoeopaths and other natural health practitioners.

MIXED METALS IN THE MOUTH CAUSE THE
SEVEREST PROBLEMS

Gold and amalgam together increase the amount of electric
current and can lead to severe heart or allergy problems in susceptible people. If a gold crown is placed next to or on top of
amalgam, it can quadruple the amount of electricity produced.
Other metals used in crowns and bridges can have similar
effects: all the metals interact with each other.

Are you allergic to other metals?

If your skin reacts to nickel, or if you cannot wear gold or other metal earrings, then the metals in your mouth could also be causing you problems. However, other metals can also cause problems in people whose skin does not react to them at all.

Mercury hypersensitivity

If you already suffer from stubborn allergies and food intolerance, then allergy to mercury is a very likely problem.

I never get any reaction when mercury is drilled out ...

Nevertheless, your general health could still be quite severely affected by it. I was in this position myself. Some people suffer a temporary setback in their condition when mercury is removed.

GETTING HELP

Metal-free fillings

White plastic composite fillings, porcelain implants for larger fillings and metal-free crowns and bridges are all available nowadays.

Can I get my fillings replaced via the National Health Service?

In Britain, National Health Service dentists will not replace fillings unless the tooth is otherwise in need of attention. Then you could ask for a white filling, but unless it is in the front teeth where it would be visible, you would have to pay privately for it.

*Could my regular dentist replace my
amalgam fillings privately?*
Possibly, but it requires special expertise. If he is inexperi-
enced in replacing amalgam fillings with white, especially in
back teeth, your own dentist may feel, as mine did, that white
fillings are not strong enough, and that by taking the amalgam
out you may lose the tooth. Ordinary dentists are caring and
competent, but because of the way they are trained they are not
fully aware of the risks associated with mercury. Mercury-free
dentists are obviously much more experienced in placing white
fillings, porcelain implants and metal-free bridges, and can
deal with problems that might worry a regular dentist and
which might therefore worry you.

BE CAREFUL
If you are having non-metal crowns or bridges fitted by an
ordinary dentist, insist that he removes every trace of amalgam
beforehand, otherwise he will almost certainly leave some in. I
have had my bridges and crowns replaced with white plastic
material, and there proved to be amalgam underneath them all
except one.

Should everybody have their amalgam fillings removed?
This is obviously unrealistic for most of us, but you may decide
not to have any more mercury amalgam placed in your mouth
in future. If you have any stubborn health problem at all, it is
worth considering mercury.

MERCURY-FREE DENTAL PRACTICES

Mercury-free dentists take special precautions to minimise the
risk of more mercury vapour being absorbed into the body during treatment. They use a rubber dam, which is a thin sheet of
rubber fixed over the lower teeth, to prevent mercury amalgam
falling into the mouth as it is drilled out.

Counting the cost

Mercury-free dental practices are all private and can be hugely expensive. Prices vary a lot so it pays to shop around. Out-of-town practices can be less expensive.

TESTING FOR MERCURY TOXICITY

Mercury-free dental practices usually offer testing. Again, there is great variation in the prices and in what they offer—from about £40 upwards for testing and a report on their findings, giving their recommendations and estimated prices for each tooth.

Urine test for mercury retention

Mercury is a cumulative poison. If you excrete less than is normal it means that mercury is building up in your body.

Sweat test for mercury

This has been known to produce false negatives, it did for me.

Blood test for mercury hypersensitivity

When London immunologist Dr Don Henderson was given the job of testing for mercury sensitivity in fifty people, forty of whom had some kind of health problem, he approached it with some scepticism. But to his great astonishment:

- 75 per cent had some sensitivity to it.
- 50 per cent were moderately sensitive.
- 20 per cent proved to be highly sensitive to it, and once it was removed much of what he saw was 'like Lazarus arising from the dead!'

It was reported in the London *Daily Mail* that one of his patients, an eleven-year-old boy, mysteriously lost the use of his legs and became confined to a wheelchair. It happened soon after his first amalgam filling was placed, and once it was removed he recovered completely and went back to playing football again!

Since Dr Henderson's work was published, the British Society for Mercury-free Dentistry has been overwhelmed with enquiries. It has also increased concern among many dentists.

Where can I get Dr Henderson's test?
See Useful Addresses. The test is expensive, but can be useful to convince yourself, your family, your employer or your doctor.

DETOXIFY WITH THE HAY DIET

For best results you also need a cleansing diet to help get rid of the mercury which remains in your body. Holistic dentists often also recommend vitamin and mineral supplements.

Little improvement?

Are you keeping strictly to the Hay diet? This is an essential backup. If you have had some fillings removed but there are still plenty left, it may just be that you have not yet lost enough mercury to feel the difference. Apparently some people have to have most, if not all of the mercury removed before they improve.

- Smoking interferes with the way the body processes mercury.

Removing mercury is just part of a comprehensive health improvement programme. It cannot be expected to solve every problem by itself and you may still have to explore other avenues. Nevertheless, you will not have wasted your money. Removing mercury certainly lightens the toxic load and eliminates a potential source of trouble in future.

Mercury and me

When I was tested I proved to have chronic low-level mercury toxicity. I found this term somewhat misleading in that it led me to believe that mercury was not as big a problem as I thought. I had no idea of the serious nature of chronic low-level mercury toxicity. Getting rid of the mercury was a huge relief to me. Natural healing is progressing very much faster now; the improvement is continuous and very impressive. It can apparently take a lifetime to eliminate mercury from the system completely, so that means a lot more improvement to look forward to!

Fruit and mercury

For many years I could not take fruit at all, it always caused a flare-up of candida. Things improved dramatically once I began having the mercury removed, but I could not take it freely until every trace of metal had been removed from my mouth.

MERCURY SYMPTOM GUIDE

Alzheimer's disease. Mercury is the metal found in the highest concentration in the brains of people with Alzheimer's disease. Mercury removal has been known to produce considerable improvement. It has even been known to reverse the condition completely, but mercury is not the only cause of Alzheimer's disease.

Candida. If candida is resistant to diet and other treatments, mercury is likely to be the underlying cause.

Hair loss. Thin hair is commonly found to thicken once mercury is removed, and even baldness has been known to improve.

Immune disorders. Mercury is a constant burden on the immune system and can therefore exacerbate immune disorders like M.E. and chronic virus infections, candida, allergies and food intolerance. I have found, almost without exception, that the people I encounter who are desperately ill with these conditions have a large number of amalgam fillings. The more different metals there are in the mouth, the worse the problem.

Low body temperature can sometimes respond to mercury removal.

Kidney disease. Kidney function can become severely impaired.

Raised white blood cell count. Constant exposure to mercury stimulates the body to produce more white blood cells in an effort to defend itself.

Leukaemia can sometimes be considerably relieved by mercury removal

Hodgkin's disease may also respond.

Mercury can be involved in auto-immune disorders: rheumatoid arthritis, ulcerative colitis, Crohn's disease and lupus erythematosis, because mercury bonds to protein molecules in the blood which the immune system then mistakes for invaders.

Tiredness, chronic fatigue. Mercury combines with oxygen in the blood, reducing the amount available to produce energy.

Failing eyesight. Many people report a drastic improvement in their vision after mercury is removed. Immediately after having three small fillings replaced my own long-distance vision improved remarkably. On testing I could see two more lines of letters, so now my optician is investigating mercury!

• The short sight which comes from hardening of the lens as we grow older cannot be expected to improve.

Diabetes. Mercury can inactivate the insulin molecule.

Food intolerance. Allergic sensitivity decreases once mercury has been removed.

Short-term memory problems. My own short-term memory

and overall mental function has improved more than I could ever have hoped. Now I can dial a whole telephone number from memory, instead of having difficulty remembering just three digits at a time!

Sore, irritable bladder. Removing mercury can bring relief. This is what finally cleared it up for me.

Travel sickness. This commonly improves. Now I can travel long distances by coach for the first time ever.

Universal reactors. These are the people who react to practically everything—every system of their body is affected. Many have mercury and a large assortment of other metals in their mouth.

It's All in Your Head by Hal Huggins further explains mercury toxicity and gives much excellent information about nutrition.

The British Society for Mercury-free Dentistry and the British Homoeopathic Dental Association practise mercury-free dentistry. See Useful Addresses.

NEW LIFE FOR SUE WITHOUT MERCURY

I had always been so fit. I'd served in the army and the police, I'd been a Russian linguist and a financial adviser, I'd always had such a bright mind. The trouble started when they pumped me full of antibiotics after an operation for sterilisation. I became so ill afterwards, with so many different symptoms, that I could hardly get out of bed, yet the doctors could not help; I couldn't understand it. I felt desolate, hopeless, and desperately afraid I might have some terrible life-threatening illness. I had thrush, too, and I was very overweight although I ate very little. I had no energy, I was living in a mess, and I had two small children.

Most distressing to me was the state of my mind. I had no clarity of thought, I just couldn't think straight. I couldn't remember anything for long, I completely forgot large chunks of the past, and I was sure I had Alzheimer's disease. I was always vaguely anxious and depressed over nothing, I would worry about every decision I made, panic and lose my grip. And I suffered like this for four whole years, always depressed and often desperate. *I searched the self-help books for answers but found none, never any mention of mercury.*

I was overjoyed to learn about candida, but although the treatment did help, I was never totally convinced I would get better until I had my first amalgam filling replaced. It was when Jackie told me how having the mercury removed from her teeth had solved more problems than all the other treatments put together, and when she sounded so much better, that I decided to go for it. The dentist I found understood: he had suffered kidney problems himself until he had the mercury removed.

I had twelve amalgam fillings; some of them were huge and blackened and they ran together along my back teeth. The test for electric currents went right off the scale. The dentist wore a mask and I wore goggles, and a mask over my nose which delivered fresh air to me from outside. He began by removing the largest fillings first and I felt better straight away after the first one was replaced. Then, as the others came out, I slimmed down from a size twenty to a size sixteen without really trying. I was still eating plenty, just keeping to a natural diet, and I'm still losing weight, almost down to a size fourteen now.

After every session I felt reborn, but three weeks later I would come down to earth again with a bump; the reactions were not pleasant but they soon passed. My head cleared first; my thinking processes have sharpened to an amazing extent. As a financial adviser I would tell people what to do, then worry and panic afterwards thinking I might have given the wrong advice, but now my confidence has returned. My memory has come back, I can remember the past and make decisions again without worrying about them. My heartburn cleared right up too, and saved me a fortune on digestive enzymes. My skin cleared, the thrush has gone, and so has the terrible constipation. They all disappeared straight away and my energy came flooding back.

Being so ill, and having the children to look after, I could never keep to my anti-candida diet as I would have liked. I was never able to give up sugar completely, nor keep strictly to a natural diet, not until I had the mercury removed. But now that my will-power has returned I manage the diet much better. After the last filling was removed I was on the ultimate high, so much energy—yet my appetite decreased. I live on a mountain, and I can walk up again, no problem. And last but not least, sex was always a chore, but not any more, our sex life is great, fantastic. Now my husband has an appointment with the dentist, he wants his fillings replaced too!

And if you are thinking all this is psychosomatic, let me tell you I had no real faith in any of this to begin with, but I was desperate enough to give it a try. I've always hated going to the dentist, but I would say to anyone, whatever you have to go through, it's worth it, just get it out of your head! The money I spent having mercury removed was nothing compared with the total expense of all the vitamin supplements and candida remedies I took over the years. It's an investment!

Having candida has forced me to take responsibility for my health; it still flares up a bit if I am careless with the diet, but I don't even miss the sugar now: it tastes disgusting, I can hardly believe it. One square of dark organic chocolate does what three bars of milk chocolate used to do for me. Now I make all our treats from The Stamp Collection Cookbook *(no wheat, no cow's milk), it's brilliant and we all enjoy them just as much.*

Useful Addresses

Action for M.E. and Chronic Fatigue
PO Box 1302, Wells, Somerset BA5 1YE
Tel: 01749 670799
www.afme.org.uk
Helplines. Information, and a very helpful magazine. Information on local contacts and self-help groups.

The Royal London Homoeopathic Hospital
Great Ormond Street, London W1N 3HT
Tel: 020 7837 8833
Temporarily operating from Greenwell Street, W1W 5BP
Great Ormond Street reopens end of 2004
NHS help for candida, food allergies, M.E. and any other problems. GP referral required.

The Breakspear Hospital,
Hertfordshire House, Wood Lane, Paradise Estate, Hemel Hempstead, Herts HP2 4FD
Tel: 01442 261333
www.breakspearmedical.com
info@breakspearmedical.com
Day and out-patients only. They have a guest house for people who live far away. Treatment for candida, allergy, food intolerance, chemical sensitivities and chemical poisoning. A private hospital but approx 20% of their patients are funded by the NHS.

The Institute for Optimum Nutrition
13 Blades Court, Deodar Road, Putney, London SW15 2NU
Tel: 020 8877 9993
www.ion.ac.uk
email: info@ion.ac.uk
Send £2 for a register of Nutritional Therapists or ring to locate a local nutritional therapist. A lively and helpful colour magazine available by subscription. Home Study Courses in Nutrition. This is also a training school for Nutritional Therapists.

British Acupuncture Council,
Park House, 206 Latimer Road, London W10 6RE
Tel: 020 8964 0222
Fully trained and qualified acupuncturists.

NHS acupuncture treatment
This is available from some hospital pain clinics, some physiotherapy departments and some GPs, otherwise treatment is private.

General Council and Register of Naturopaths
Goswell House, 2 Goswell Road, Street, Somerset
BA16 OJG.
Tel: 01458 840072
Closed on Wednesdays, open Saturdays 9 a.m.–1 p.m.
Ring to find your local practitioner.

National Institute of Medical Herbalists
56 Longbrook Street, Exeter, Devon EX4 6AH
Tel: 01392 426022
www.nimh.org.uk
email: nimh@ukexeter.freeserve.co.uk
Send large SAE plus postage payment for 150g in weight.

Society of Homoeopaths
4a Artisan Road, Northampton NN1 4HU
Tel: 01604 621400

Bristol Cancer Help Centre
Grove House, Cornwallis Grove, Clifton, Bristol BS8 4PG
Tel: 0117 980 9505 (help line)
0117 980 9500 (centre information)
www.bristolcancerhelp.org
Natural approaches, including diet. Information on nutrition and cancer available from help line database.

The Hyperactive Children's Support Group
71 Whyke Lane, Chichester, West Sussex PO19 7PD
Tel: 01243 551313
Open 10am–1pm most weekdays
www.hyperactive.force9.co.uk
email: hacsg@hyperactive.force9.co.uk

Foresight (The Association for the Promotion of Preconceptual Care)
The Paddocks, Godalming, Surrey GU7 1XD

Natural Justice
Bernard Gesch, 1 Trinity Hall, The Gill, Ulverston, Cumbria, LA12 7BJ

The National Society for Research into Allergy (NSRA)
PO Box 45, Hinckley, Leicestershire LE10 1JY
Tel: 01455 250715
email: nsra.allergy@virgin.net

The Vegetarian Society
VSUK, Parkdale, Dunham Road, Altrincham, Cheshire WA14 4QG
Tel: 0161 925 2000
www.vegsoc.org
email: info@vegsoc.org
You can send a stamped addressed envelope for their excellent information sheets.

USEFUL ADDRESSES

Health Interlink
International House, Unit B, Asfordby Business Park, Welby,
Melton Mowbray, Leics LE40 3JL
Tel: 01664 810011
www.health-interlink.co.uk
email: info@health-interlink.co.uk

Doctors specialising in allergy and nutritional medicine

In Britain, doctors who specialise in nutritional medicine and
who practise desensitisation to foods and airborne allergens are
now available through the National Health Service, if you can
get funding from the GP or via the hospital specialist. It can be
dificult to obtain. A very few of these doctors work in the NHS.

If you are paying privately, you can consult a private doctor
without a GP referral if necessary. Most are happy to discuss
the problem on the telephone first.

British Society for Allergy and Environmental Medicine,
PO Box 7, Knighton, Wales LD7 1WT
*They have a list of doctors with a special interest in allergy and
nutritional medicine.*

Action Against Allergy,
PO Box 278, Twickenham, Middx TW1 4QQ
Tel: 0208 892 2711

Biolab Medical Unit,
The Stone House, 9 Weymouth Street, London W1N 3FF
Tel: 020 7636 5959
www.biolab.co.uk
*Private consultations in nutritional medicine. Laboratory tests
for body levels of vitamins, minerals, essential fatty acids—
and much more. A private laboratory but patients can also be
funded by the NHS.*

British Society for Mercury-free Dentistry
221 Old Brompton Road, London SW5 0EA
Tel: 0207 373 3655
This is an expensive test currently costing £200 including tele-phone consultation. A kit for taking blood can be obtained by ringing the Society. Blood can then be taken at your local GP surgery.

UNITED STATES OF AMERICA
American Preventive Medicine Association
459 Walker Road, Great Falls, VA 2206
Tel: (800) 230 2672
A register of practitioners sympathetic to natural medicine.

The CFIDS Association of America
PO Box 320398, Charlotte, NC 28222 0398
Help for chronic fatigue.

The Feingold Association of the United States
127 East Main Street, Suite 106, Riverhead, NY 11901
Help for hyperactivity.

The Food Allergy Network
10400 Eaton Place, Suite 107, Fairfax, VA 22030 2208
Tel: (703) 691 3179
email fan@worldweb.net

DAMS Dental Amalgam Mercury Syndrome
Theresa Kaiser MA, PO Box 64397, Virginia Beach,
VA 23467
Tel: (800) 311 6265
Patient support organisation.

Other therapies

Local Hospital Physiotherapy Departments
Aromatherapy is becoming more widely practised by hospital physiotherapists, especially in connection with chronic pain, but whatever the problem, it is worth enquiring.

Local Colleges of Further Education
Some now run courses in holistics, including aromatherapy, reflexology, body massage and Indian Head Massage. Supervised treatments given by students are at much reduced prices.

Here's Health
Popular and very helpful monthly magazine which supports the approach taken in this book. Available from larger newsagents and by ordering through local newsagents.

Natural Health Exhibitions
These make a good day out and they open your eyes to the tremendous variety of the healing arts. There are stands representing every possible therapy and plenty of experts to talk to. One example is the Vitality Show at London Olympia each spring. There are lectures, workshops, cookery and fitness demonstrations, and bookstands specialising in complementary medicine. They are usually advertised in *Here's Health* magazine. Many smaller exhibitions are organised locally.

FOOD SUPPLEMENT COMPANIES
All food supplement companies are user-friendly and will answer any queries. You can order by telephone using a credit card. Their mail order services are fast and efficient:

Quest Vitamins Ltd
Venture Way, Aston Science Park, Birmingham B7 4AP
Tel: 0121 3590056
Free information line staffed by qualified nutritionists.

Lamberts Healthcare Products
1 Lamberts Road, Tunbridge Wells, Kent TN2 3EH
Tel: 01892 554313
They supply Zincatest, a taste test for zinc deficiency.

Cytoplan Ltd
Unit 8, Hanley Workshops, Hanley Road, Hanley Swan, Worcestershire WR8 ODX
Tel: 01684 310099
Natural food state vitamins including vitamin C. Linseed (flax seed) oil. Loose psyllium husks.

Spatone Iron +
Freepost Spatone, Trefriw Wells Spa, Trefiw, Snowdonia, North Wales LL27 0BR
Freephone: 0800 7311740
Liquid Iron, non-constipating.

Biocare
Birchwood House, Briar Lane, Croydon, Surrey CR0 5AD
Tel: 0180 777 3121
Vitamin and mineral supplements for hyperactive children, also acidophilus powder.

Metabolics Ltd
5 Eascott Common, Devizes, Wiltshire SN10 4PL
Tel: 01380 812799
www.metabolics.co.uk
Wide range of herbal tinctures, nutritional supplements, anti-fungal preparations and products pecially formulated for easy tolerance. Private consultations also available.

Further Reading

The Hay diet

The Hay Diet Made Easy, Jackie Habgood, Souvenir Press, 1997.

Food Combining for Health, Doris Grant and Jean Joice, Thorsons, 1984.

The Food Combining Diet, Kathryn Marsden, Thorsons, 1993.

Food Combining for Life, Doris Grant, Thorsons, 1995.

Food Combining, Tim Spong and Vicki Peterson, Prism Press, 1993.

A New Health Era, Dr William Howard Hay, Harrap, 1933.

The Superfoods Diet Book, Michael Van Straten and Barbara Griggs, Dorling Kindersley, 1992.

VIDEOTAPE
Light as a Feather, Linda Robson and Patrick Holford, Vision Video Ltd, 1994.

Recipe books

The Food Combining for Health Cookbook, Jean Joice and Jackie LeTissier, Thorsons, 1994.

Food Combining for Vegetarians, Jackie LeTissier, Thorsons, 1992.

The Stamp Collection Healthy Eating Cookbook, Terence Stamp, Ebury Press, 1997.

Sugar-Free Cooking, Elbie Lebrecht, Thorsons, 1994.

Sugar-Free Desserts, Drinks and Ices, Elbie Lebrecht, Faber & Faber, 1993.

Low blood sugar

Low Blood Sugar, Martin Budd, Thorsons, 1984.
Hypoglycaemia, Marilyn Light, Keats, 1983.
Hypoglycaemia: A Better Approach, Dr Paavo Airola, Health Plus, USA, 1977.
Hypoglycemia: The Disease Your Doctor Won't Treat, Jeraldine Saunders and Dr Harvey M. Ross, Pinnacle Books, USA, 1980.
New Low Blood Sugar and You, Carlton Frederick, Perigee Books, USA, 1985.
Sugar Blues, William Duffy, Warner Books, USA, 1975. *About sugar itself.*

Candida

Candida Albicans. Could Yeast Be Your Problem?, Leon Chaitow, Thorsons, 1991.
Beat Candida Cookbook, Erica White, 1993, available by post. Tel: 01702 72085.
Candida Albicans, Gill Jacobs, Optima, 1990.
The Missing Diagnosis, Dr Orion C. Truss, 1982. Publisher: Box 26508, Birmingham, Alabama 35226.
Tissue Cleansing Through Bowel Management, Bernard Jensen, Bernard Jensen International, USA 1991. Available through The Fresh Network, 01353 662 849.

M.E. and chronic fatigue

Link to Life, Kevin Mulhern (ed.), Boxtree, 1994.
M.E. How To Live With It, Dr Anne McIntyre, Thorsons, 1989.
Feeling Tired all the Time, Dr Joe Fitzgibbon, Gill & McMillan, 1993.
Tired of Being Tired, Michael A. Schmidt, Frog Ltd, California, 1983.
From Fatigued to Fantastic, Dr Jacob Teitelbaum, Avery, USA, 1996.

FURTHER READING

Allergy and food intolerance

Not All in the Mind, Dr Richard Mackarness, Thorsons, 1976.
Food Allergy and Intolerance, Dr Jonathan Brostoff and Linda Gamlin, Bloomsbury, 1989.
Asthma Epidemic, Dr John Mansfield, Thorsons, 1997.
The Migraine Revolution, Dr John Mansfield, Thorsons, 1986.
The Pulse Test for Allergy, Dr Arthur F. Coca, Max Parish, 1959. Reprinted by St Martins, USA, 1996.

Allergic children

Hyperactive Child, Janet Ash and Dulcie Roberts, Thorsons, 1986. *Natural recipes*.
Hyperactive Child, Belinda Barnes and Irene Colquhoun, Thorsons, 1984.
Hyperactive Children, Shirley Flack, Bishopsgate Press, 1987.
Are You Allergic? Dr William Crook, Professional Books, USA, 1975.

Food and mood

Not All in the Mind, Dr Richard Mackarness, Thorsons, 1976.
Food, Teens and Behaviour, Barbara Reed, Natural Press, USA, 1983.
Mental Illness—Not all in the mind, Patrick Holford (ed.), Institute for Optimum Nutrition, 1995. *A very useful booklet*.
Mental Health and Illness, Carl Pfeiffer and Patrick Holford, ION Press, 1996.
Nutrition for Your Nerves, Dr H. Newbold, Keats, 1993.
Inner Harmony Through Bach Flowers, Sigrid Schmidt, Time-Life Books, 1997.
Vitamin B3 and Schizophrenia, Dr Abraham Hoffer, Quarry Health Books, Quarry Press, 1998. Address: PO Box 1061, 240 King Street, Kingston, Ontario, Canada. Email: info@quarrypress.com *Contains medical data*.
Optimum Nutrition For The Mind, Patrick Holford, Piatkus, 2003.

General information about the effects of food

Principles of Nutritional Therapy, Linda Lazarides, Thorsons, 1996.

The Food Factor, Barbara Griggs, Penguin, 1986.

Naturopathic Medicine, Roger Newman-Turner, Thorsons, 1984.

The Whole Health Manual, Patrick Holford, Thorsons, 1988.

The Saccharine Disease, T.L. Cleave, Keats, 1974.

Complete Nutrition, Dr Michael Sharon, Prion Press, 1989.

Nutrition and Physical Degeneration, A. Weston Price, Keats, 1990.

Diet, Nutrition and the Prevention of Chronic Diseases, World Health Organisation Technical Report Series no. 797. Report of the WHO Study Group 1990, HMSO.

Evening Primrose Oil, Judy Graham, Thorsons, 1984.

The Fats We Need to Eat, Jeanette Ewing, Thorsons, 1995.

The Whole Health Manual, Patrick Holford, Thorsons, 1988.

The Consumer Guide to Vitamins, Angela Dowden and Graham Lacey, Pan Books, 1996.

The Zinc Solution, Dr Derek Bryce Smith, 1987.

The Food Factor, Barbara Griggs, Penguin, 1989.

Food and Healing, Anne Marie Colbin, Ballantine Books, 1986.

A Time to Heal, Beata Bishop, Penguin, 1996.

Complementary medicine

Homoeopathy: Medicine for the 21st century, Dana Ullman, Thorsons, 1988.

Medicines, Dr I.K.M. Morton and Dr J.M. Hall, Bloomsbury, 1997.

Naturopathic Medicine, Roger Newman-Turner, Thorsons, 1984.

Principles of Nutritional Therapy, Linda Lazarides, Thorsons, 1996.

Cancer and Leukaemia: An Alternative Approach, Jan De Vries, Mainstream, 1988.

Aromatherapy Oils

The Directory of Essential Oils, Wanda Sellar, C. W. Daniel Company Ltd, 2001.
The Art of Aromatherapy, Robert Tisserand, C. W. Daniel Company Ltd, 1977.

Mercury toxicity

It's All in Your Head, Hal Huggins, Life Sciences Press, USA, 1989.
'Menace in the Mouth?', Jack Levenson, Green Library, 1999.

Other self-help books

The health section of any bookshop, and all public libraries, carry a large selection of books on the natural approach to every illness. You will find there are so many things you can do to help yourself that you will never run out of ideas.

To obtain the books listed above

American books not available in UK bookshops can be ordered by post from:

The Nutricentre, 7 Park Crescent, London W1N 3HE
Tel: 0207 436 5122
Open 9 a.m.–7 p.m. Monday to Friday
10 a.m.–5 p.m. Saturday
www.nutricentre.com
email: enq@nutricentre.com.

Or from
Revital, 35 High Road, Willesden, London NW10 2TE
Freefone: 0800 252 875
www.revital.com
email: info@revital.com

They may also be obtained by post from Internet bookshops
such as
UK: www.amazon.co.uk
USA: www.amazon.com

Out of print books may be obtained from your local library, or
will be listed on their computer. If they do not have a particular book they may be able to order it for you from another
library.

Bookfinder service: Many W.H. Smith bookshops have special
bookfinder computers which show you a list of books on any
given subject on the screen. You can also order any book by
telephone: 0345 581549 (Monday to Saturday, 10 a.m. to
7 p.m.) for the price of a local call. It will be sent to your
local branch for collection.

Mail order: Waterstones Bookshops operate a mail order
service from all their shops.

More Help for Candida

In view of the enormous number of problems with Candida and gut infections that have brought to my attention since the first publication of this book I thought it would be helpful to update my research and experience in this special appendix.

CANDIDA AND OTHER GUT INFECTIONS

Microscopic intestinal parasites and harmful bacteria such as E.Coli can mimic the symptoms of candida, and they can all thrive together in a dirty, sticky, sluggish gut. Millions of us unknowingly harbour these parasites, especially now that we travel abroad so much more. The antibiotics and steroids in meat also lower our resistance to parasites and gut infections of all kinds. Organic meat is best.

CHRONIC CONSTIPATION

As explained on page 66, highly processed foods like sugar and white flour lack the fibre to move through the gut properly and they turn into a sticky paste which adheres to the bowel wall, forming a thick layer of debris along its length. This gradually slows down the natural peristaltic movement of the colon and can practically inactivate it over the years. It creates the perfect breeding ground for candida, parasites, and bacteria, and they far outnumber the friendly bacteria which help to keep candida under control.

Irritable bowel

People who have loose stools or irritable bowel may also have a thick rubbery coating along the bowel wall and they too may benefit from colonic irrigation. Colonic therapists are always willing to discuss the problem over the telephone.

You can now find out exactly what is going on in your gut

There are now private laboratories which can analyse the stools. They identify the harmful bacteria and parasites and assess the degree of candida overgrowth. They send you a collection pot and you send them the stool by post. See 'Health Interlink' under 'Useful Addresses'.

I was greatly relieved to have my own stool tested and horrified at the high level of candida overgrowth after so many years of dieting and anti-candida medication. It also revealed what I could never have suspected, that I was full of E.Coli bacteria *plus* parasites. My dirty gut had obviously rendered the medicines practically ineffectual.

Laboratory tests are not absolutely essential

The money I spent on the tests could have paid for three of the colonic irrigation treatments described below – and they should clear the infections out of the gut anyway. But I had the money for them at the time and I was glad to be able to identify the problem.

Colon cleansing with herbs

A good colonic therapist recommends a herbal colon cleanse to soften the contents of a loaded bowel before treatment. Make sure you get a colon cleanse, before you begin. Not all colonic therapists work like this and the irrigation will not adequately release the accumulated debris without it so, enquire what the treatment consists of before you decide, or you could be wasting your money.

Find a colonic therapist who is also a qualified western Medical Herbalist if you can

See The Association of Master Herbalists under 'Useful Addresses'.

You may find that a herbal colon cleanse is all you need to clean your bowel

But be careful: Colon cleansing tablets or packs can sometimes be extortionately expensive. Food supplement companies and herbalists can usually supply them at a reasonable price. See 'Useful Addresses'.

Colonic irrigation accelerates recovery from severe chronic candida

If candida keeps coming back despite an anti-candida diet and if no amount of medicine will dislodge it you may benefit from colonic irrigation.

This is what you can expect:

- The tube is introduced to the body by a greased metal speculum which is then removed leaving the tube inside the body – not painful, just momentarily uncomfortable.
- Warm filtered water is gently introduced into the gut, through a double rubber tube, about a litre at a time, from an overhead tank, where the water temperature is thermostatically controlled.
- The tube is then clipped to keep the water in the colon for a few minutes while the abdomen is gently massaged to distribute the water along the colon, and to soften and loosen the sticky deposits on the bowel wall. This is important.
- Then the water is gently released through the other side of the double tube and goes straight into the sewage system.

- This process is repeated several times and the whole treatment will take at least and hour. There is no smell and very little discomfort.
- There is a glass connection in the tube so that both you and the therapist can see what comes out of the bowel. Candida can come out in large blobs of yellowish mucus. Softened bowel debris, which has been stuck to the bowel wall for a very long time, can sometimes come out as a black tarry substance.

Many candida victims complain of mucus leaking from the anus

I had twelve colonics at three to four-weekly intervals. Candida mucus was present in all but the last of them, the twelfth was clear. After the first colonic I felt so wonderfully clean and fresh inside that I knew I was on the right track. After three treatments I could eat fruit in moderation after twelve years without it. But the old bowel debris did not begin to come out until the fourth treatment. That encourage the bowel to work by itself, so the constipation began to improve. It usually takes about three colonics before achieving a really good result. I now consider I wasted my money on anti-candida medications over many years because I was so unaware of the vital importance of cleaning the gut from the beginning.

- Colonics cost from £45 per treatment. Out of town therapists may be less expensive.

Is colon cleansing the complete answer to candida

Not necessarily because if you have chronic candida the infection will have already spread from the gut and invaded other tissues throughout the body. Aromatherapy oils, especially tea tree, can be highly effective against systemic candida, especially since they are absorbed through the skin and not the gut and go straight into the tissues. As explained below, it takes regular treatment, over weeks or months to obtain the best results. So while you still have problems it is wise to keep to the diet and carry on taking acidophilus.

Sceptical?

'Tissue Cleansing Through Bowel Management' by Dr. Bernard Jensen contains many colour photographs of the results of bowel cleansing!

AROMATHERAPY OILS FOR CANDIDA

Before I began training in aromatherapy I understood it to be no more than just a scented massage. Nothing could be further from the truth. Aromatherapy is an ancient and modern system of medicine, now scientifically validated and currently used not only by aromatherapists, but by at least 1,500 French GPs.

- During the 1920s Gattefosse, a French perfumier, badly burned his arm whilst working in his laboratory and immediately thrust it into a vat of Lavender oil. To his great astonishment it healed extremely rapidly, without scarring. This led him to investigate the healing properties of essential oils.
- During the middle ages, many of those people in Europe who used essential oils on a regular basis managed to escape the plague.

Aromatic oils were not used therapeutically in Britain until the late 1950s. The rest of the world has been using them for centuries, frankincense, myrrh and spikenard to name but a few. Tea tree oil is a more recent introduction.

Again the great advantage of essential oils to a food intolerant person is that they go in through the skin, avoiding gut reactions.

Tea Tree Oil for Candida

Tea tree oil is strongly antifungal, antiviral, and a powerful immune stimulant. I have found that the most potent effects are obtained from essential oils by self massage. Dilute one or two drops in 5–10 ml carrier oil, such as grape seed or sweet almond oil, both of which are available from supermarkets and health food shops. Then you can massage *the whole amount* into your skin, preferably after a bath or shower, leaving a minimum of 5 days between treatments. The oil prolongs the invigorating effect of a shower for several days. Do not shower for another 12 hours so as not to wash the oil off. If you dislike the smell of tea tree, remember it only lasts for about half an hour at the most.

Essential oil of Lavender is also antifungal and antiviral, and is used in the same dose. Avoid it during the first three months of pregnancy. It may sometimes cause drowsiness in people with low blood pressure. Incidentally it is also a surprisingly effective natural sedative, antidepressant and tranquilliser.

These are both extremely powerful oils so be careful not to overdose on them. Dropper bottles vary, and sometimes the oil comes out too fast. If you drop it into a small bottle or plastic medicine cup first before adding the carrier oil, then you can throw the essential oil away and start again if you release too many drops. Just one drop too many can prove too much. An extra drop of tea tree oil keeps me awake all night. One drop too much lavender oil gives me a headache!

I have found that Julia Lawless Essential Oils come with the easiest droppers.

Both tea tree oil and lavender oils have a stunning array of additional properties, and they work! See 'The Directory of Essential Oils' by Wanda Sellar.

Index

bacon 28, 137, 144, 156
bananas 23, 26, 27, 31–2, 103, 121, 146
barley 29, 38, 47–8, 89
beans 26, 29–31, 66, 103, 105, 123, 127, 148, 157
beanshoots 29, 126
beansprouts 30, 60
bedwetting 152
beetroot 60, 122
belching 126–7
bingeing 33, 36, 94, 102
biscuits 23, 28, 37, 48, 53, 93, 179
bladder problems 46, 48
bloating 25, 43, 109, 116, 127, 129
blood pressure 15, 44, 190, 195, 219
blood sugar levels 43, 149, 172, 175, 185–6, 188–9, 200
    effects 142–3, 166, 182
    high 112–13
    low (hypoglycaemia) 13–14, 22, 33–4, 38, 43, 50, 69–105, 123, 164, 174, 177
        causes and symptoms 78, 79–82, 135–6, 218
        effects 37, 139, 167–8, 181
        remedies 74, 76–7, 97–105, 120, 139, 192
body odour 50, 110
bowel cancer 56, 67
bowel problems 46, 51, 66, 115–16, 129, 152, 218
bran 29–30, 67
bread 16, 21, 26, 29, 38, 43, 47–8, 88, 107, 118, 120
    see also gluten
bread, white 28, 53, 57, 63, 88–9, 96, 137, 179, 206
bread, wholemeal 28, 31, 101, 103, 173–4, 189
breakfasts 22, 31, 58, 64, 122
breast pain 198

buckwheat 47, 120
burning sensations 111, 116, 133
butter 28, 31, 105, 122–3

caffeine 88, 92, 95, 98–101, 169
    effects 69, 78, 80–1, 83–4, 87, 90, 94, 100, 102
cakes 28, 48, 53, 63, 125, 179
calcium 54, 57, 157
cancer 17, 42, 49, 54, 57–8, 115, 190, 198–9, 220
candida 13–14, 34, 38, 77, 106–33, 144, 187–8
    anti-candida diets 36, 118–28, 168, 231
    causes 98, 113–14, 135, 218, 227
    remedies 13, 17, 101, 107–8, 108, 118–33, 199, 230
    symptoms and effects 35, 107, 108–13, 139, 163, 165–6, 168, 207
caprylic acid 130
carbohydrates 53, 66, 92, 173–4, 200
carrots 29, 101, 103, 120, 122
catarrh 12, 133
celery 29, 101, 120, 122
cellulite 17, 37, 39, 41, 190
cereals 25, 28, 31, 89, 156
cheese 21, 26, 29, 31, 41, 66, 103, 115, 118–19, 148–9, 179
chemical sensitivity 107, 113, 218
childbirth see pregnancy and child-birth
children 46, 57, 89, 94, 108, 144–5, 151–62, 182, 195, 201, 206, 216
    diets 155–7
chocolate 23, 28, 37, 41, 42–3, 53, 93, 96, 133, 185–6, 231
    effects 86, 100, 125, 132, 137, 142, 185–6

INDEX